MW00414263

THE
YOGA
OF
LOVE

*Based on Sri Aurobindo's
Synthesis of Yoga*

TALKS AT CENTRE

3

M. P. PANDIT

PUBLISHER:
LOTUS LIGHT PUBLICATIONS
P.O. Box 2
Wilmot, WI 53192 U.S.A.

First U.S.A. edition February 21, 1982

Published by Lotus Light Publications
by arrangement with Sri M. P. Pandit

Cover Design: Paul Simpson

ISBN: 0-941524-16-7

Library of Congress Catalog Card Number 81-86373

CONTENTS

1

DIVINE LOVE

We now begin the subject of subjects—Love. Before we start studying Sri Aurobindo's exposition of the role of love in the Integral Yoga, I would like to give you an idea of how the subject of love for God has been dealt with in the Indian tradition.

When these traditions were formed, scriptures were handed down orally. There was no system of writing and even when writing was systematised, there was no paper. Things were written on palm leaves and other leaves which could stand the test of time. So, necessarily, the communication had to be as brief as possible. The teacher would explain a certain theme and conclude in an abbreviated statement. This condensation of a theme called a *sutra* in Sanskrit is inadequately translated in English as an "aphorism". In India, as Sri Aurobindo has observed somewhere, the passion to develop a science of epitomisation, of condensation, was such that it was said that if one could manage to leave out even a single syllable from the aphorism, he felt as much joy as in the birth of a son!

The aphorisms of Patanjali on yoga are so brief that unless somebody expounds what is behind the words, what is the content, they are very difficult to understand. That is why many scholars who are not familiar with the background of Indian thought have been misled.

Now, coming to our subject, the most celebrated treatise on Divine Love in India is by the sage Narada, who is counted among the sons of the Creator, Brahma.

He begins in the style in which all the Sutra treatises, the aphorisms, begin. "Now, therefore, we shall expound Divine Love. What is Divine Love? That, verily, is of the nature of the supreme love of God." Love of God, that is devotion, is a supreme love, not the kind of love that we are familiar with on earth, which depends for its existence upon certain antecedent factors, depends for its growth on the fulfilment of desires. It is something supreme, something transcendent. So, that love of God which is uncaused, which does not depend on other factors, that is true devotion.

And what next? Narada says, "In its own intrinsic nature, Divine Love is immortal." Unlike human love which is mortal because it depends upon factors outside itself, Divine Love is immortal. It is a self-existent, self-awakened love; it has no end. There may be a stopping in its manifestation due to various reasons, but this fount of love from within has no end, no death, no ceasing. That is why it is immortal.

Further, if devotion is supreme love, if that supreme love is immortal, what are its effects? The fourth Sutra elucidates, "Gaining that, man becomes fulfilled, becomes immortal, becomes fully satisfied." Man is satisfied, he becomes conscious of something immortal in him, so that he is no longer afraid of death, he is fulfilled. His own existence, he feels, has attained its purpose. When one is aflame with love for God, when one is consumed in its flame, there is nothing else that one can desire. Man feels then that life has reached its acme—he looks for nothing else, thinks of nothing more.

The next Sutra says, "Attaining that he has no more desire for anything. He has no grief; he grieves for nothing. He hates not; he does not rejoice in anything else, nothing else holds his attention; he has no

eagerness for anything." The usual vital propulsions
for activity and movement—desire, enthusiasm, enjoyment, hatred of the enemy—which normally move a
person into activity, no more exist for him.

These are the negative signs; and what are the
positive ones? The Sutra explains, "Realising that, he
becomes intoxicated." It reminds us of the famous lines
of Sri Aurobindo, "I have drunk the Infinite like a
giant's wine." He is intoxicated. He is rooted, he does
not flow out; there is no tendency to spread out—not
only physically but even mentally and emotionally.
He is rooted to the object of his love, and a whole empire
of joy is in his soul. A key expression in the Upanishads
around which whole philosophies have been erected
speaks of such a one as *atmarama*, one who delights in
the Self.

But Narada warns, "This love, this devotion is not
lust, because it is a form of renunciation." This is an
intense love, an intense preoccupation with the delight
of the Self, but its nature is not of lust, of conquest, of
domination, but of renunciation. This is the difference.

Narada goes on to describe other features into
which I will not take you. He next discusses the characteristics of this intense devotion, this intense love. He says
there are many viewpoints regarding this; many sages
list it differently. He refers to a sage, Parashara, who
describes this love and devotion as: "Activation, self-
employment in worship and adoration". Another sage,
Rishi Garga, says, "It is attachment to sacred talk
of God." There is yet another sage, Shandilya, as
prominent in his field as Narada, who says, "Whatever
the occupation, it must be without prejudice to one's
delight in the Self." But Narada himself, after mention-
ing these differing views, records his own estimate,

and he says, "The essential characteristics are consecration of all activities by complete self-surrender to Him,
and extreme anguish if He were to be forgotten." Posi-
tively, its characteristics are: complete self-surrender
within, and an exhaustive, comprehensive self-consecration in all activities. Negatively, they are what the
Mother calls a sense of suffocation—like a fish out of
water—, what Narada terms anguish, if God were to be
forgotten.

The ancient Indian tradition speaks of nine forms
of devotion. They are at once movements for the expression of devotion and feeders for the flame of Divine Love.
They are:

> *Shravana*—listening; listening to the glories of God,
> listening to the legends and histories of God-
> men, receiving the divine vibrations through
> the sense of hearing.

> *Kirtana*—laudation; praising of the Lord from the
> depths of one's heart.

> *Smarana*—remembrance; whatever one is doing,
> whatever the movement, to remember, and to
> offer.

> *Padasevana*—physical service; physical service im-
> plies consecration at the physical level. Not
> merely a theory in the mind, not merely an
> attitude of the heart, but a rendering on the
> physical plane of one's submission and conse-
> cration.

> *Archana*—worship; physical worship, maybe
> through flowers, incense, water, leaves and the
> like, or an inner worship—visualising the Lord
> in a form and a pouring out on the physical

plane of one's emotions, the best of oneself, before it.

Vandana—bowing down. Bowing down is not merely a physical act of folding the hands or bending the head. It is the end-result of an inner attitude of submission.

Dasya—Taking up the attitude of a servant; this means a readiness to serve, whatever be the nature of the service demanded by the Divine.

Sakhya—a readiness to assume any attitude called for by the Divine; the attitude may be one of a servant or servitor but as the Mother has said, there is also the attitude of a friend, of a comrade. The Divine reveals Itself in many aspects and the devotee has to be ready to meet and greet the Lord in any poise.

Atmanivedana—complete self-surrender in all the parts, on all the planes of the being, at all times, in all places.

These are the nine limbs of Divine Love. Then, further, Narada asks himself if one's experience of Divine Love can be described. He says, "It cannot be described". When the sap of the Divine Love courses through one's veins, can one really describe it to another? He says, "When a dumb man tastes a delicacy, can he really describe what he tastes, what he feels? This as such is indescribable." Then he adds, "Attaining That, one hears only That, one talks only (of) That, one thinks only (of) That." When one does nothing else, then it is a sign that he is consumed by the Divine Love.

Narada next discusses the various types of God-lovers. He analyses, following the *Gita*, that there are four main types of those who aspire and seek for Divine Love. First, there are those who are in distress—physical, or psychological—and they seek the help of God.

There are those who seek material welfare, material benefits from God—that also He grants. This is the second category.

Then there are those who know something of God— maybe by hearing, or by reading, or by experience— and they want to know more. And in their seeking for that knowledge, their devotion grows. So the third category is of those who are ever desirous of knowing the Lord.

In the fourth category are those who are the knowers of God. The *Gita* says that they are dearest to Him. By "a knower of God" is not meant a philosopher, one who knows the metaphysics, who has studied the treatises and knows the definitions of the Absolute, the Immutable and the Formless, but one who knows God intimately.

And now we have arrived at the point where we can take up Sri Aurobindo's exposition of Love.

In the *Gita* it is said that he loves God most who knows Him. What is the relation between knowledge and love? If we take knowledge in the sense of a mental appreciation, of a mental analysis of what God is and what He is not, what leads to God and what leads away from God, that is not the kind of knowledge that is related to love. But the knowledge that lands me in the lap of God is that which makes me feel that God is within me, that God is around me, that I have no existence apart from God, that I breathe and live because of God. When that knowledge fills my cells and flows through my veins, can I help vibrating with love for that Divinity? Love is the crown of knowledge. True knowledge ends in love, even as real, wide, spontaneous love which is either vouchsafed to one or springs from the fount of the heart leads one to the perception of the existence of God everywhere. Love opens many windows on the Reality that is God; one cannot escape perceiving God when one is filled with love for God. Even as knowledge culminates in love, love leads to an integral knowledge.

2

LOVE AND THE TRIPLE PATH

It has been the traditional attitude in Indian sprit-uality to look upon the path of knowledge as exclusive, but the adherents of the path of love, too, look upon theirs as the one true path, and those who tread the path of works look askance at the followers of the other two. Of these three, the arrogance of those who take up the path of knowledge is insufferable, especially of those who follow the path of pseudo-knowledge.

There is a well-known story of Vivekananda when he was very young. In one of his visits to his master, someone told him that across the river there was the house of a very great scholar, a renowned man, and it would profit him to call upon him and learn from him what he had to say about God. Out of sheer curiosity the young man went to the scholar's house, but found that he had gone for a bath in the river. He waited, and in the meanwhile, he stepped into the library of the great man and found against the wall many almirahs stacked with books. He handled a few of them and put them back. By that time the celebrity arrived, and after due introductions, the young man asked, "Sir, have you really read all these volumes?" The scholar replied, "What doubt is there, my dear boy? Of course I have read them." Then Vivekananda said, "But I have found some volumes with uncut pages." The man could not bear to be found out. He said, "Someone had borrowed those books and didn't return them, so I replaced them with new copies."!

Sri Aurobindo makes certain good-humoured remarks on this pride of the intellect which looks down upon humility and the humble approach of the devotee to the Lord. He points out that while it is true that knowledge helps one to scale the altitudes of the spirit, to know more and more of the heights of the being, it is equally true that it misses something of the largeness of the heart, the profounds of the emotions which open the gates to the sweet intimacy of the Divine. There is also a tendency among those who follow the path of knowledge to give a false status of superiority to the impersonal over the personal aspect of the Divine. They have it that what takes form, what expresses itself in a personality is limited, and what breaks out of the form—the Infinite, the Impersonal, the Qualityless, the Void—is the real truth, the Absolute.

But, if you ask the adorer of form, the devotee who meets the Divine in its sweet personality, the personality that pours out love, he will not trade any one realisation of his with a hundred realisations of the *jnanin* or the knower. In fact, he looks down upon the dry-as-dust knowledge of the intellectual. He proclaims that the true taste of bliss is in love. The dry aridities of knowledge do not satisfy him. Sri Aurobindo is careful to point out that while the God-lover is right in what he says, he too misses the truth. The love that is enlightened, the love that is lit up by the lamp of knowledge is far more satisfying than an ignorant love or a love that is at the mercy of circumstances. Love that is founded on a true understanding, is more rounded, more full.

In his Integral Yoga, Sri Aurobindo reconciles the conflicting claims of the three paths of knowledge, love and works in the Indian tradition. He points out that if we admit that the expression of the Divine in man is not limited to one power, one faculty, there will be no difficulty. In fact, all of us are aware that there are in us the elements of knowledge, action and love expressed by the mind, the will, the heart. Now these are the three modes of self-expression of the Divine in each man.

It is all right to start from any one of these points where one is most awake. By nature, one may be more developed in the mind. So he starts with a study of what others have said on the basis of their experience and speculation. Thus he starts on the way of knowledge. But as he goes on, not only understanding the truths that are taught, but assimilating them in his own consciousness and translating the knowledge to the best of his ability in day-to-day life, he begins to understand the Divinity as expressed in his depths or on the heights of his being, there is an awakening of love, of devotion for the Divine that he has begun to know. Knowledge culminates in love; true knowledge leads to true love for the Divine, otherwise it remains a purely philosophical and speculative knowledge. Knowledge that is true to the consciousness, knowledge that is assimilated in one's consciousness is bound to awaken love as its consequence. And once knowledge is crowned by love, the will automatically and spontaneously blossoms forth in pouring out the various powers and energies of the being in consecration to the Divine who is experienced through knowledge and through love.

So even though one starts on the path of knowledge, if sincerely pursued in a comprehensive and not in an exclusive way, the path branches off into the path of love, and leads to the path of works. Ultimately, knowledge, love and works all combine to produce a rich and many-sided realization.

Similarly, one may start with the path of devotion. One has a spontaneous welling up of feelings and emotions for God, and for him or her who embodies God for him. He turns towards anything that recalls the divinity to him. All this is an indication that that part in him is ready and he has to make that the focal point for the initial concentration of all his energies, powers and faculties and make a beginning on that path. Gradually, however, as the devotion spreads, stabilizes itself, deepens into adoration, and adoration melts into love, he begins to realize that the Divine whom he worships, the Divine whom he waits upon in the solitude of his heart is not confined to his initial conception. More and more aspects of the Divine begin to reveal themselves to him and a natural knowledge begins to dawn about the integral nature of the Divine. The key is, indeed, love, but as the key turns and the door opens, it reveals treasures of knowledge that add a certain comprehensiveness and width of outlook.

And if that knowledge—that the Divine is spread all over—, if the warmth and the ebullition that result from love for the Divine are true, the devotee cannot remain satisfied with bottling up those experiences in himself. He delights in consecrating all of himself—thoughts, feelings, emotions, activities, even physical and vital movements to God. There is an effortless channelling of the dynamic will in the path of works. The more he works in this spirit of love with the background of this knowledge of the comprehensive manifestation of God, the richer becomes the quality of the works that are done.

So also, even if one is not gifted with the clarities of the mind, with the clarities of knowledge, even if he finds the doors of the heart locked and finds himself

apparently incapable of any warmth of feeling towards
the Divine whom he does not see physically, he can, if
he has the will to turn his life Godwards, take to the
path of works. Whatever activities are assigned to him
by circumstances, he turns them into channels for the
outpouring of his consciousness towards the Divine.
He does the work in the spirit of disinterested service,
and in the measure of the sincerity he brings to bear
on his practice of the yoga of works, there is a loosening
of the heart-strings. He begins to feel a certain warmth,
a certain closeness to the Master to whom he offers his
work. There is an automatic growth of inner relation,
and with the formation and growth of this inner relation
there is a growth of sentiment, a growth of devotion
which he begins to cherish. That opens the fount of love,
and then as his will gets trained in selfless consecration,
his heart backs up the endeavour by adoration and
warmth of sentiment developing into love. He feels
and begins to cognize the different features of the presence of the Master. So, bit by bit, he begins to understand and respond to the presence of the Divine in him
and around and above him.

Thus, from whichever point one starts,—works,
love, or knowledge—properly pursued, each path
gathers up the realisations of the other two paths, and
in the end the seeker of the Integral Yoga finds that all
of them combine to produce a magnificent orchestra
of harmonies.

This forms a kind of introduction to Sri Aurobindo's
treatment of the way of love and emphasizes that this
way of love is not an exclusive path. It combines in
itself, if not in the beginning, but as it develops, as it
culminates, the gains of the path of knowledge and the
path of works. From the divine standpoint, all are equal.

It is only from our petty, human standpoint, dominated by the one-sided knowledge of the mind, that one may appear superior and another inferior. But in the Divine scheme of things, as you know, there is nothing superior, there is nothing inferior. All has its role, its legitimate work; it all depends upon the spirit in which we look at things. Everything has its place when looked at in the proper perspective. Love, knowledge, action—these are the three fundamental elements in the being of man, linking him with the Divine. The Divine expresses Itself in all the three and all the three can be utilized as channels of approach to the Divine. If all are combined with a judicious selection and assimilation, the result is quicker and richer.

(FROM QUESTIONS & ANSWERS)

Is it possible to begin with all three paths at the same time?

Yes, that is precisely what the Mother wants us to do. When a person turns to spiritual life, it means that he has developed to a certain standard. He is aware of the many parts of his being—he is aware of his will, he is developed enough in the mind and certainly, he is conscious of his heart, his feelings. And in the beginning itself, if one has this integrated approach, there is a harmonious growth in yoga. I think it was in one of his letters to Champaklal that Sri Aurobindo says that by going to the Himalayas and doing sadhana there, you may develop powers of meditation, trance, the capacity of going into yourself, but you are lost to the larger and vaster realization of the Divine in the universe. So if, when we start, we start with the consecration of our energies in disinterested work, and at the same time develop the finer emotions and turn them Godward, linking our work to the flow of our emotions, and at the

same time take care to refine our mind, clarify our understanding, guard ourselves from the error of offering our
works and emotions to inferior powers and instead
make them over to the true Divine Reality, we save ourselves from many pitfalls. And each element helps and
guards the others. It is a quicker, and I might say, a
more natural process of spiritual evolution, more in
keeping with the divine intention in the cosmos, than the
several exclusive pursuits. It is for the sake of clarifying
things that Sri Aurobindo says that one starts at any
point, but if one can, one should certainly start at all
points.

   We in the twentieth century know that man does
not have a single personality. Each one is aware of the
multiple personalities in him, and unless the multiple
personalities develop, man does not turn to yoga, to
spiritual life. A person turns to spiritual life when his
evolutionary development has reached a certain mini-
mum multi-facetted pattern around the soul. The soul is
awake on many fronts; apparently it may not be so, but
with a slight cultivation, the soul reveals that it thirsts
for knowledge, it flows with love, and it surges in will-
ings. That is the Mother's distinctive contribution: we
must start in a large way. Though the advance may
appear slow in the earlier stages, the results are far more
satisfying, and the response it evokes, the comprehensive
nature of the working of the Grace that is present,
makes up for everything and much more.

   Regarding the world situation, they are talking so much
about disasters, that people will be wiped out and that great
cataclysms are coming. But it seems to me that it won't happen
like that. It's as though the world has gone down the wrong
road and it's backing up to go down another road, and it seems
to me that the disasters will come more in the consciousnesses of

people who are not developed. But somebody who is developed will have enough to eat and enough to wear and he will be all right...

For those who are developed, physical disasters don't have that much relevance—whether they have enough to eat and drink or not. For them there is no problem.

For the rest, I think the stage is past when there could be a possibility of a great fall-back of evolutionary nature casting aside man on the roadside and going on to develop a new species. That stage is past; higher levels of consciousness have already descended and are integrating themselves with the earth and I do not at all expect any such kinds of disasters or catastrophes as would hold back the progress of mankind. The aberrations you see are very much on the surface.

Also we must know that the mass media which dish out reports of world events, world trends are given to exaggerate small, inconsequential things. And today, when there is such a shortage of newsprint that certain newspapers and journals have had to close down, nearly one or two columns are devoted, with abominable photographs, to a new phenomenon that has started all of a sudden in the United States—young men stripping themselves and running through crowded thoroughfares, naked. Well, if one is completely naked, there is some artistry about it at least, but these, to make themselves more grotesque, have their headgear and shoes and stockings on. Naturally, stripping in public is against the law, against decency. When the police pursued them and tried to arrest them, there were fist-fights, there was stone-throwing, and the climax was reached when the Vice-President of the United States, due to preside

over a ceremony, was greeted by these young men and
women. They call it streaking—they do not allow themselves to be caught, they rush away. And within three
days of the appearance of these phenomena in the United
States, French youths started imitating them near the
Eiffel tower in Paris.

Now this is put down as a sign of youth unrest,
youth ferment. Accepted, but as if to prove it is not so,
the older people have also started it and because they
can't run, they have given it a different name. They call
it snailing. We wonder what kind of a world we are in.
These are things to be laughed at; if you make much
of them, then they tend to stick. If they are looked upon
as some sort of aberration, and you don't take notice
of them, they will just die down.

But, after all, are we not really making too much of
youth unrest? Is it really confined only to the youth?
The unrest is spread over all the layers of society; at
every stage, at every level there is an imbalance calling
for redress, calling for readjustment. And at the bottom
of it is the refusal of man to keep pace with the advanc-
ing pace of Nature in evolution. Nature calls for a certain readjustment, reformation, a giving up by each individual, of the egoistic standpoint and an enlarging of
the individual consciousness to keep abreast of the
enlarging movement of the universal consciousness. As
long as men as individuals, and men as members of
collectivities, refuse to move away from their old primitive moorings to their selfishness and ego, these things
will continue. And it is to demonstrate the absurdity
of the situation that all kinds of phenomena are being
heaped upon us. These incidents are symptomatic of a
certain imbalance; by themselves they are oddities, but
they are to be taken as signposts of the stagnation that

has taken place. The human vitality, the human force, takes all kinds of abhorrent forms because right and legitimate avenues are denied to it by the obstinacy of man.

    ...in **Savitri,** *Death says to Savitri, "Know also that in knowing thou shalt cease to love, and cease to live..." and Savitri answers, "When I have loved for ever, I shall know"...*

Death knows that he will lose his empire when love comes into its own, because love is eternal. True love knows no end, it takes one to the heart of things, to the soul of things. That is why Death wants to mislead Savitri by telling her that when she really begins to know the truth, when she begins to analyze, she will find love just melting away. Love has no real existence, it is fashioned out of the hopes and imaginations of men. As her knowledge grows, she will see how transient love is. But she replies that this is not so, as she loves more and more, as she gets nearer to the heart of love she will know everything. There love and knowledge melt into one, and the crux is in the culmination of love, even as the acme of knowledge is the realisation of a total oneness—a oneness of being, oneness of life, oneness of mind, oneness of everything. The more one loves, the more one identifies oneself with the object of love, and becomes one with it.

    So this realization of oneness is the final stage of the growth of love through all the vicissitudes of its evolution; the Supreme Love culminates in a total identity of the lover and the loved.

*   *   *   *

    The Samadhi is a profound concentration of the vibrations of the physical embodiments of both the Mother and Sri Aurobindo. By going physically near

2

to those subtle-physical vibrations, many sense an
opening, many feel a nearness to the Mother which
they do not feel otherwise. Many feel openings in the
different centres of their being when they go there
physically, because they are very much conscious of
their physical bodies themselves. Also, there lie the
physical bodies of those whom we love, whom we
cherish. We don't need to go there for any experience;
we go because somebody whom we have loved is there,
the body is there which we have worshipped, cherished
and loved. So it is with a spontaneous feeling of love
that we go, not necessarily to gain a spiritual experience, not to effect an opening in ourselves, though all
those things can happen. There are many who do not
go, they don't need to go. But there are those who
need to. Then there are those who go even without
the need, it is a spontaneous movement.

But the fact remains that on the physical plane,
for those who live in the physical consciousness normally, physical symbols, physical images, icons, form
some sort of links with the supraphysical realities.

*   *   *   *

Love for the Divine is incomplete unless you
love the Divine in others also. The Mother says it is
meaningless for sadhaks to quarrel with each other
and then say they love her. She says, "If people love
me, they have to love me in others also". So true love
for the Divine is incomplete unless it flows to the
Divine in the universe, to the Divine in those around
you. Whether they respond or not, it shouldn't really
matter, but on our side, on the side of those who are
awakened and who house that flame of Love, there
should be a continuous emanation only of forces and

vibrations and thoughts of love. Love does not care whether it is recognized, love is not less if it is not recognized. Certainly, if love is responded to, it grows— that is another matter, it is a positive aspect. But one should love to radiate more and more, wider and wider. Only that way can love be established and stabilized and helped to grow in oneself.

3

THE MOTIVES OF DEVOTION

I welcome you all to this house where I have
learned what it is to love. It is from here that I first
received the vibrations of love from the Mother. This
house has certain historic associations not merely for
me because I lived here with my teacher for more than
twelve years, but for all who are connected with the
Mother. For it was given to the owner of this house,
who belonged to one of the most aristocratic families
of Pondicherry, to put the first garland on the Mother
when she landed in Pondicherry. Many things have
happened since then. The Mother has paid visits to
this house, though not after I came to stay here. She
had asked my teacher to stay here, and it so happened
by a series of circumstances, that I also found myself
living here. It is from the terrace of this house that I
had the first glimpse of the Mother's white aura, of
which I have spoken to you in one of our talks. It was
at the door of this house that the Mother stopped her
car and gave the flower "surrender" to my teacher
when he was very ill. It was here that I used to stand
for years together at about a quarter to four when the
Mother was driven to the tennis court and she would
bestow her tender smile on me as she passed. My
whole life has revolved and has been revolving around
her smile of Grace.

My sadhana, my way of yoga has not been one
of knowledge, though it might appear that I am a
man of knowledge. Nor has it been one of works, though

there is, apparently, no dearth of works in my life, but essentially mine is the way of love—of devotion, adoration, surrender. When I was asked, in my very early years here, what boon I would ask of the Divine, were I given the opportunity, I remember having said, "Devotion for the Mother". And in one of my first interviews with the Mother, when there was mention of it, I told the Mother that there was not enough of spontaneous devotion in me, though mentally I had a great and deep regard. She just asked, with half a smile, "Oh, isn't there?" And since then I have not known a moment when there has not been that spontaneous flow of love for the Mother, for anything associated with the Mother, for anything that bears the name of the Mother. Having had this experience for some decades, it did not require much persuasion for me to accept her dictum that love is the greatest power on earth. That love is the easiest gate to open to the Divine has been said by many, many mystics all over the world, but I do not know if anyone has said that love is a power, and the greatest power at that. In fact, from our human point of view, love is considered to be a weakness, a sentiment which people of power, of might, of strength look down upon as the prerogative of weaklings. Perhaps this can be said of what passes for love among human beings, but even there the Mother's outlook is quite different. She would not condemn human love as most of the ascetic traditions in India and elsewhere do. She has always held that human love is the first imperfect expression of the true love which is trying to manifest on earth. Bound as we are in egoism, ignorance and false-hood, it takes the form of a self-regarding love—some call it lust when it is mixed with physical passion, but whatever it is, it is self-regarding. It may start with a movement of self-giving to the other person, but sooner or later it is accompanied by a subtle demand that there should be a response, a give and take, otherwise they complain of a one-way traffic.

This is what the Mother calls bargaining. This habit of bargaining, that starts and continues on the human level, prolongs itself even in our relationship with the Divine in the earlier stages or even later, depending upon when the process of purification and catharsis is started.

But human love is a step to Divine Love. The Mother affirms that one who is not capable of human love finds it extremely difficult to open to the Divine Love. For the first indispensable step in both is the willingness, the capacity to give oneself—here in the lower stage, to give oneself with the expectation of getting something in return, whereas in the higher form, it is a self-giving with no expectation. Whether it is love between a man and a woman, between a mother and her child, or between members of the same family or the same society, these are only variations in degree of human love. The human element of expectation or demand is there. But in the Upanishad, it is unequivocally declared that one must love another not because it is one's wife, or because it is one's husband, but because of the Self within—the capital Self, mind you, not the egoistic self or the desire-self. There is one Divine, stationing itself in me, stationing itself in you or in another. When we come into contact with another, the Self in one body recognizes itself in the other body and calls. If there is not that immediate call, it only means that there are still many layers or veils of ignorance to be pierced. When these veils are not there, when the Self recognizes and sends out its vibrations, calling another, there is what is called affinity.

Love is the greatest factor for unity. We speak of world unity, of collectivity, collective consciousness, gnostic consciousness, gnostic community—which is held as the ideal before Auroville, as it was held before the Ashram for a long time—but how can this community come into being unless each member opens himself to Divine Love? And this Divine Love cannot take root, cannot sprout unless the element that constricts, the element that narrows—the ego—is eliminated. One has to die to oneself before one can be reborn in God's love.

This is the importance of love. We may know, we may work, but unless our hearts are widened enough, our emotions trained to flow truly, widely, unless we are able to identify ourselves with those around us fully, not keeping any reserved areas for ourselves—unless all this is done, a real collectivity of the spiritual type cannot come into being. That has been the Mother's message. Indeed there are many aspects of her teachings. But if I were asked to sum up her teachings in one word, to sum up her life in one word, I would reply, "Love, love and love". It is with a great thrill that I open the third part of *The Synthesis of Yoga*,—the Way of Love,—in order to be able to share with you all my little experience of love, my little knowledge of love, the drop of love that meant an ocean for me and has changed the whole character of my life and the direction of my career.

In our last session we saw that it is possible to strive and arrive at God by means of works alone, by means of knowledge alone, by the way of love alone. But all these are partial realizations. For a seeker of the Integral Path, Sri Aurobindo emphasizes that all the three should converge. You may start from any point that you are attracted to. If your mind is developed, if to have a knowledge of God attracts you, no doubt you will start with knowledge. You begin with the discipline of the mind where you first separate things that are impermanent from those that are permanent. Then you withdraw your consciousness from the impermanent and identify yourself with what is permanent and eternal. This is called the method of discrimination. Gradually you detach yourself from that which passes—the passing show as it is called— and center your consciousness on the Eternal, the Permanent, the Absolute Truth, the Divine. Once you do that, once you allow your consciousness to be so affected, to be filtered through that experience, then every action and reaction has to proceed from this center of consciousness which has been shifted from the outside to the inside. You raise the frontiers of your mind above the narrowness of the creeds and dogmas of religion and philosophy to which men normally are accustomed, recognize that nobody can have a monopoly on Truth, open the windows of your mind to the fresh winds of thought and development and receive the breath of knowledge from wherever it comes. Finally, what is most important is to translate this knowledge into practice. Otherwise it remains, as Sri Aurobindo has described in another connection, only on the top shelf where nobody touches it. It has to be brought down into life. If you are mentally convinced that all is Brahman, all is God, it will not do for you to keep it as a mental formula; it has to be

rendered into your day-to-day life. You have to allow
it to colour your feelings, your emotions so that you
do not look upon X, Y and Z as people other than
yourself, but as portions of God, the same God of
whom you are a portion. The consequence is a natural
flow of charity, an easy understanding, a spontaneous
harmony, a welling out of love for others. It will not
do to parrot formulas of the knowledge left by our
ancient seers. The knowledge has to be translated, you
have to express it in your day-to-day movements.
Your actions become channels not only for the radi-
ation of knowledge, but also means for the stabilization,
for the establishment, for the confirmation of that
knowledge in your own consciousness. The result of
this double operation—having the knowledge in the
mind and working out that knowledge in the ways of
will, action—is the development of a natural love for
the Divine, for God wherever you turn. So even if
you start with knowledge, you culminate in love, love
of God everywhere.

There are those who are dynamic, who have got
a will to work. They don't care for knowledge, and
they say their hearts are dry, they have nothing to do
with love, but they work. They are blessed with plenty
of vitality and energy, which they are willing to dedi-
cate to the Divine. Well then, as Sri Aurobindo says,
start there; that is Nature's indication to you of where
to start. You place your will at the disposal of the
Divine, make yourself an instrument, offer your work
to the Divine. The test of true offering is only to work
and not to care for the result, not always to have an
eye on the distant result, the fruit. Once you offer
work to the Divine, it is the lookout of the Divine
what the results are. Once you start doing disinterested

service, the will gradually gets identified with the higher Will of the Divine, and instead of your offering to the Divine, being a servant of the Divine, you become an instrument of the Divine. It is a divine Energy that flows through you, it is a divine Will that presides over your will and acts. This sincere dedication, wholesale identification with the Divine leads to a complete identification of your consciousness with the consciousness of the Master, of the Mother who receives your offering, your consecration and works through you. You become a child of the Mother—from being a servant of the Divine, an instrument of the Divine, a channel of the Divine, you become a child of the Divine. You become identified with the Divine, and when you are identified with the Divine, you know the springs of your actions are in your love for the Divine. Works culminate in love.

And there is the third category of those who start with loving the Divine. They feel a spontaneous devotion for the Divine, not necessarily for God in a church or a temple. They feel the presence of the Divine maybe in a beautiful flower, in the ocean, in the horizon, in a beautiful person, in music—everywhere. There are a thousand ways in which the Divine reveals itself. You feel a spontaneous rising of the consciousness, and it expresses itself in adoration. You develop devotion for the Divine, and as this devotion grows, it flows into an outer adoration; outer devotion expressing itself in worship slowly changes into an attitude of inner adoration which continues even when you are not physically engaged in the ritual of devotion. This inner adoration, as it deepens, melts into love. There is no more the consciousness that you are the adorer and the Divine is the adored. There is total

oneness; with the birth of love, there starts the identification, the growth towards union with the Divine,
for union is the crown of love. As you love more and
more, you begin to know what you love. There is a
spontaneous manifestation of the contents of the being
that you love, and that is true knowledge. And love
cannot be bottled up. It is impossible for love of God
to be corked into yourself; it insists on flowing out—
flowing out in words, in emotions, in actions—in acts
that reach out the Grace of God, that speak out the
Love of God. Even when you start with love, the way
of love gathers on its way the gains of knowledge, the
gains of works.

So whichever way you start—knowledge, works,
or love—all the three combine. And for us who are
human beings of the twentieth century, who have
known a multiple development of personality, a many-
sided development of consciousness, it is natural to
seek an integral realization. We have, in the course
of the last two years, familiarized ourselves with the
essential concepts of the yoga of works, followed by
broad outlines of the yoga of knowledge, and now
the crowning phase is the yoga of love. It is only when
we allow our understanding of the yoga of works and
the yoga of knowledge to blossom into the yoga of
love that we shall be ready to put our first step in
what Sri Aurobindo has called the Yoga of Self-
Perfection. It is a long way still to go, but each one of
us here is fortunate in this, that each has tasted a drop
of the Divine Love that poured out through the manifestation of the Mother. Whether all who are here
have had the privilege of personally meeting and
having a physical exchange with the Mother or not,
the fact that they are here in this atmosphere which

has been charged with the presence of the Mother and Sri Aurobindo for over five decades is enough guarantee that they cannot escape the vibrations of love that are packed in this mystic community called "The Ashram" and its extension "Auroville". We know what we mean by love. At any rate in the context of yoga, we know that love is based upon the psychic principle, is based upon the principle of consciousness. What is Consciousness in the higher hemisphere— the upper half—is projected on earth as knowledge; what is Force, Consciousness-Force there, is projected here as force, strength, power; what is Existence is projected as being, matter; and what is Delight, Bliss, projects itself as love. And the seed of love—just as knowledge is embodied in the mind, power and force in the will, existence in matter—is embodied in the psychic centre, the psychic being.

We have seen in one of our talks how man first begins with a psychic essence. That essence, as one grows, becomes the psychic element, becomes a psychic entity. The psychic entity, with further development— mainly spiritual—becomes a psychic personality. And when the psychic personality arrives at its acme of development possible in the human body, it unites with the Overself, the divine representative presiding over the destiny of each individual. So the source of love is in our depths.

All religion, all spiritual life aims at establishing a bridge between man as he is and God as he conceives Him to be. Most of the religions imagine or conceive of God as a power, as some existence above. Man is a pale reflection, a tiny entity, who has to strive, to labour and arrive at God. But though religions posit an enormous distance between God and man, yoga aims to bridge the gulf and to arrive at the union of man with God. You start with the conceptions of religion as they are, but as you begin to practice yoga— the inner discipline of the expansion of your conscious- ness, of the deepening of your consciousness—you begin to realize more and more that the Divine is the highest term of your own being. When you work for God you begin to realize, as your will gets identified with the Divine Will, that ultimately in the measure in which your will becomes one with his, you become one with him. So in love; you start worshipping God— yourself the worshipper and he the worshipped—, but as the yoga of devotion develops, as the inner adoration deepens, there is neither the lover nor the loved, there is only Love. This is the function of yoga.

There are religions which conceive of God in the image of man. It has been humourously remarked that God conceived man in his own image, and man returned the compliment. He thinks of his narrow self, his way of doing things, his way of accepting things—flattery, praise, condemnation, anger—and he invests God with all these qualities, necessarily in a magnified form. God is a magnified man—he punishes, so there is fear, but he is amenable to flattery, and he will weigh the scales in your favour on the day of judgment if only you know how to flatter him. So there are psalms, there are prayers in which, after you have sinned merrily, you seek to redress the balance by lauding him, by taking his name at the last moment.

Now all these are anthropomorphic conceptions, relics of the past. Man today has awakened and he knows that what he thinks is not even the best image of himself. He himself has evolved and he knows that

these ideas and images—psychological and physical—
are primitive and he has to leave them behind. There
are philosophers who would point out to you that to
think of a personal God, to think that by worshipping
a personal God you will arrive somewhere and you
will receive his grace is another superstition. They say
God is infinite, God is impersonal, God is immutable
and it is a folly of the human mind to conceive of
the Divine in human terms. Well, if the Divine is
impersonal, certainly there is no room for love. For
what happens in spiritual life when one conceives of
the Divine as impersonal is that one stills the emotions,
keeps the mind in silence, and there is only a settling
of calm, of peace, of a deep sense of oneness. The
culmination of that movement is what the Buddha
called Nirvana—silencing of all movement and activity,
your individual world ceasing to be.

Certainly this is not the intention and purpose of
the Divine in manifesting the universe. The purpose
of man is not salvation, not escape, not Bliss, but
fulfilment of the Divine purpose on earth, in life. It is
true, there is an aspect of the Divine which is
impersonal. That, Sri Aurobindo points out, is only
to emphasize the freedom of the Divine to break out
of all the limits of formation. You think of God the
Beautiful, you think of God the Merciful—well, there
are areas of manifestation where beauty, mercy do
not apply; the infinity escapes these definitions. It was
to underline the freedom of the Divine to exceed all
formulation that the dictum of *neti-neti* in the Upanishad
—'not this, not this'—came to be. "Not this" means
"He is not only this"; it does not mean "This he is
not," it means he is much more. He is much more
than what you see, he is this plus something else. He

is this world, but he is not exhausted by this world.
If he were only this world, it would be sheer pantheism.
He is much more. One of the ancient verses in the
Veda describes that he created the world out of himself,
and exceeded it by a 'digit'. Only one-fourth is here,
three-fourths is above. I am not sure of the arithmetic,
but the idea is that he exceeds his manifestation.

There is the transcendent—the individual is a
reality, the universal is a reality—but above, there is
the transcendent. The transcendent is also a reality.
Normally the individual is shut up within himself, he
does not even have access to the divinity within him,
to the individual Divine. He has to make a special
effort or he has to be blessed by Grace to get an opening
into the universal Divine. Or he has to make an effort
by rising and shooting upwards into the transcendent.
But is it possible for an individual to realize the Divine
in all the three aspects? Yes, says Sri Aurobindo, and
that opportunity has been given for the first time to
humanity because of the manifestation in the Mother.
For the Mother combined all the three embodiments
of the Divine—the transcendent, the universal and the
individual in herself; and by so doing she gave a chance
to every individual who aspired for it to attain that
triple realization in his own life. That possibility, that
actuality has not passed with her physical passing, for
it has been established on earth as a permanent possibility for everyone who cares to seek for it—to realize,
first God within, then God around, and God above.

The impersonal is not the sole truth, the personal
also exists. If you ask a devotee who has had the realization of the Divine as a person, he will tell you that
the impersonal is only the background out of which
the personal emerges, but it is the personal form that

is paramount. It is not possible for an aspiring individual to connect himself consciously with what is impersonal, with what is infinite. Whom can you pray to if there is only an impersonal Divine, and who is going to respond, who is going to help? It is to enable the human consciousness to link itself with the Divine, to lift the human out of the present belt of ignorance, that the Divine takes a personal form. There have been various personal manifestations, which help us to concentrate and converge our movements at one point. The Divine is the Lord, he is the Master, he is the Beloved; once you have that magnet, that center of reference, the rest is a natural unfolding.

It is all right for the man of knowledge, for the *jnanin* to scoff at love and say that it is a concession to the ignorant. It is also understandable if the man of love, who knows the Divine only through love, were to condemn the man who seeks knowledge as a dry-as-dust philosopher who has only partial knowledge. Well, these are all partial truths. It is easy for us who are following the broad, many-aspected teaching of Sri Aurobindo and the Mother to appreciate the role of each path, the role of each way towards the blossoming of Divine Life. And in that blossoming, love has a capital role to play.

There are two or three other points with which I shall sum up. Even in the yoga of love, nobody pretends that everybody starts with the purest of emotions, with the purest of motives. Man is an evolving being, so first there is the lure of desire, the lure of earthly satisfaction. Man starts praying to God, thinking of God, asking of him things that he wants and the Divine gives. Until a man turns to spiritual life, every sincere prayer is answered in the terms in which things are sought. There was a sage on the western coast of India who was known—and is still known fifty years after his passing—to grant the worldly desires of his devotees. Anything one asked for—health, wealth, progeny—he would give. And when he was asked, "You are a man of God; instead of asking people to give up their desires, instead of denying them and giving them a shock and awakening them to the higher Reality, why is it that you are granting their worldly desires?" He replied, "I give them what they want so that they may begin to ask for what I want to give them."

And it is true that after the first wave of satisfaction is spent out, one begins to be ashamed of one's petty demands and starts giving up a little by little the emphasis on earthly satisfactions. There is the story of a thief who had gone to steal fruit from a wealthy man's garden. While he was busy with his operations, he was startled by the sounds of a number of people from the house rushing towards him. All ways of escape were closed. He thought for a moment and had a brain wave. Quickly he cast aside all his clothes and sat cross-legged with eyes shut. When people came with lanterns and torches to catch the thief, they only saw a holy man. So they went and woke up the owner. The owner and his wife came with flowers and incense, and bowed before him. The next morning the newspapers were full of the holy man and a whole procession of people kept coming, bowing down, offering coconuts, fruits, flowers and money. The thief was moved. He said to himself, "What is this? I am not a holy man. I am a fake. And yet the whole world is coming to pay me homage! Supposing I were really a holy man?" And that very day he changed his life; he gave up his old profession for good, took to *sannyasa,* and walked away leaving everything. A great movement of renunciation had taken place. We do not know what happened afterwards, but the moral is obvious. In unexpected ways at times, God gives you his touch.

There are so many different kinds of people at so many different stages of development. There are some people who have reached a certain stage of development and the ego has served its function, but there may be others who are less developed in which case it may still be necessary for the ego to function......?

The ego has certainly a part to play in the development of the personality. Ego is Nature's device to have a point around which the flow and flux of life can be organized so that there is a point of individuality. Once the point of individuality has been formed, once the point of reference has been built up and one is habituated to referring everything to it, that is the point when it may be said, "Ego was the helper, ego is the bar." The ego is a help to many, but when one arrives at the threshold of spiritual life, the ego becomes a bar. In the normal day-to-day life, the ego is a help, but when it comes to spiritual life, the ego becomes an obstacle. The ego has to be progressively thinned out until it disappears. After all, the ego is only a deputy—when the deputy goes, it is the Principal, the real center of God, the soul, that comes forward.

You need not preach the removal of ego to those who are still wedded to the ways of ignorance, who have not yet arrived at a stage in their evolution when they are impelled to take a leap into a Godward life. It is for those who aspire for a higher life that the ego has to be eliminated. For a politician, for a military commander, for a surgeon, a certain self-confidence, a certain egoistic self-regard is an instrument-ation that Nature develops and through which it acts. Even the Divine acts through the ego of certain instru-ments as long as they can serve only from that level.

Will there be a marked worldwide change if the ego begins to go from many people?

It is true that nowadays there is a mental recogni-tion all over the world that the ego or self-interest should cease to be the final arbiter of things. Things must be looked at and decided from a larger and a more universal standpoint. To that extent there has been a gain, there has been progress, there has been a recognition of the necessity of pushing the ego back. But there is not yet enough sincerity in the people who matter to give up that ego. Each one expects the other to give up his ego. The Mother says, if we do not learn, if we refuse to learn, Supernature has its own way of shocking us into sanity, the crash of cir-cumstances will force human beings to think differently, to see differently and to act differently. It is not a question of not knowing, it is a question of wanting to practise what we know, a question of sincerity. All of us who are gathered here know exactly what is right, what is the thing to be done. The question is whether we are sincere enough to translate into practice what we know. There may be a hundred extenuating circumstances for our not giving up the ego, but that is what holds us back.

4

THE GODWARD EMOTIONS

We have seen that in yoga it is any one power or a number of powers of one's consciousness that are utilised as the means to establish contact and develop a relation which will culminate in a union with God. We saw last time how in the yoga of knowledge one starts with one's mind, with the faculty of thinking, discriminating. In the yoga of works, one starts with the will, the will to consecrate and unite one's own will with the divine will and work as its instrument. And in the yoga of devotion—which is the theme of our present series of talks—it is the emotions that are the means used to approach God.

Any human relation that is possible with the Divine is taken up, developed and intensified, so that through that relation the human consciousness may be cultured and developed to be capable of an ultimate identity with its objective, the Divine. There are any number of possible relations with God, but in many religions, especially of the Semitic origin, it is the fear of God that dominates, and I would say, vitiates the intimate relation that man can have with God.

The explanation for this perverse twist in the human approach to God can be explained historically in this way: originally when the intelligence of man was not as developed as it is today, man tended to conceive of a superior being in control of the universe, a superior power which could influence life—both his own and in the world. He imagined a power or a number of powers which could promote his prosperity as well as push him down the road of adversity. And he invented ways and means to propitiate these powers so that they could further his ambitions and desires, and he also found out ways and means—prayers, petitions, supplications—to avert the wrath of God from his destiny.

The root and the basis for that fear is the conception of sin. It is regarded in certain religions that man is originally tainted with sin, and God is conceived as somebody who can be bribed to hold back the consequences of sin from those who know how to propitiate him, and who condemns others who are not able to do so to an eternal hell. Of course, in the Indian religions also there are the conceptions of heaven and hell, but they are regarded not as products or the result of some original sin with which man is born, but as reward and punishment for the good and bad deeds done by him with his own free will. Whatever the reason, the element of fear of God is one of those hostile intrusions in the cosmic scheme.

I remember Mother saying somewhere that fear is totally alien to the divine intention. Even as falsehood, so too fear was not originally foreseen when the movement for manifestation gathered momentum. Fear was a totally unexpected intervention precipitated by the asura, the titan, the anti-Christ. Where there should be only love, where there should be only a flow of sweetness, fear has been introduced and there is an aversion, a shrinking, a withdrawal. However, now that it is established as a part of the evolving world in ignorance, it has to be faced and eliminated.

The first conception and formation of fear as one of the ruling factors determining our relation with the Divine gradually gave way to the conception of God as a ruler—a ruler of law and righteousness, and one who awards the fruits of one's labour—a little bit of an improvement on the original conception. Gradually the idea of good and evil, virtue and vice took root. The idea that punishment is meted out by God has still remained. Everyone should know that God is not there to punish—man punishes himself enough. Every day of his life, when he errs, when he allows his consciousness to deviate from the Right, from the Truth, his consciousness goes down and grooves are formed in his being through which his wrong movements flow helplessly. Is that not enough self-punishment? Man punishes himself out of ignorance, and he can cease to punish himself in the measure in which he comes out of the belt of ignorance.

In the Indian religions, instead of the fear of God it is the lure of heaven and the fear of hell that has come to dominate. Exaggerated stories of saints in paradise, of the fires of hell, have worked havoc in the natural growth of the human soul in the East. There are even traditions which don't believe in God at all, but only in heaven and hell after this life. If God and the gods exist, they are a part of this scheme of Paradise and Hades. Life came to be looked upon as an opportunity to win entry into one and avoid precipitation into the other.

We have been speaking of the somewhat primitive conditions of the evolution of religion, because it is in religion that devotion largely took root. Yoga takes over from religion this contribution of devotion for God, but purified from many of its grosser elements.

In yoga, particularly in the yoga of devotion, one takes up any relation that permits an interchange, an outflow of one's emotions. There is the conception of the Fatherhood of the Divine, as one who protects, as one who saves, in whom one can trust, whom one approaches with the devotion and the love of a child. Closely allied to the conception of the Fatherhood of God is the Motherhood of the Divine. The Divine is conceived and experienced and realised as the Mother, the Divine Mother-Soul, the Divine Creatrix of all, to whom the child-soul comes for succour, for nourishment, for growth, for receiving the warmth of her love. And, Sri Aurobindo observes that the Mother-soul wishes that the child should so approach her. Whether the reason is spiritual, religious, ethical or what is called mundane, the Divine Mother welcomes the child and takes it as an opportunity to pour out her heart of love on the child. That is the essence of the relation between the Motherhood of God and the childhood of the human soul.

The Divine is also looked upon as a helper, as a friend, to whom one looks up, on whom one relies. After all, as the Mother asks, is not the Divine your best friend, one who does not ask you to be other than what you are and still wishes you to arrive at the utmost fulfilment of which you are capable? In this concept of the Divine as a friend, there is a certain basis of equality which is foreign to many religions. It is in yoga, and in certain Eastern religions based upon love, that one approaches God in terms of equality, as a friend and a comrade, and throws off all inhibitions. No doubt, when one deals with the Divine

in embodiment as a friend, there is always the danger
of the human relation of friendship covering up the
awareness of the infinite greatness of the Divine.

Doubtless most of you have read the Gita, and
have read how prince Arjuna, who was the companion
of Lord Krishna—the charioteer of the human soul—
moved with him in utmost terms of friendship and
equality. And the legend runs that when Krishna
was discoursing to him on the battlefield where Arjuna
had lost his nerve and conjured up several reasons
why he should not fight, the Lord counselled him to
fight, and Arjuna asked him, "How am I to believe
that you are the Lord, and not just Krishna my friend?
May I see your cosmic form?" The Lord agreed but
said, "You cannot see my cosmic form with your
physical eye," and gave him the inner eye, the Divine
eye to behold the divine vision that was being revealed
to him.

With this inner eye, Arjuna sees before him a
thousand-armed, a thousand-headed cosmic form rang-
ing from the heavens to earth, spread everywhere.
He sees the millions of soldiers who are standing for
battle passing through his mouth, being also masti-
cated by his teeth, blood flowing on all sides. He sees
also all the past rishis and sages and kings and
monarchs passing through his mouth and he is
staggered. He realises suddenly how lightly he has
treated Krishna; he awakes to the enormity of the
fault that he has committed and overcome with the
utmost humility, he prays to the Lord.

"Salutation to Thee a thousand times over and
again and yet again salutation, in front and behind
and from every side, for Thou art each and all that is.

Infinite in might and immeasurable in strength of action, Thou pervadest all and art every one. For whatsoever I have spoken to Thee in rash vehemence, thinking of Thee only as my human friend and companion, 'O Krishna, O Yadava, O Comrade,' not knowing this Thy greatness, in negligent error or in love, and for whatsoever disrespect was shown by me to Thee in jest, at play, on the couch and the seat and in the banquet, alone or in Thy presence, O faultless one, I pray forgiveness from Thee, the immeasurable. Thou art the father of all this world of the moving and unmoving; Thou art one to be worshipped and the most solemn object of veneration. None is equal to Thee, how then another greater in all the three worlds, O incomparable in might?"

It is a classic description of the possibility of human relation veiling the divine relation. As these relations are being formed, they express themselves in various ways. In Indian scriptures there are nine different ways in which one seeks to express one's love for God, and they are: first, *hearing*—hearing of the glory of God, constantly listening; then *chanting*— chanting his glory; *remembrance*—remembrance of the Lord, not only during the period when one worships, but even at other times; *service*—service of God in himself and in the world; *adoration*—the ritual of adoration; *salutation,* which means much more than the physical bringing together of the palms. It means the assembling of all the life-energies and focussing them in a gesture of greeting and surrender to the Lord. Then, *obedience*—obedience to the will of God; *comradeship*—of which we have spoken just now; and finally a full, unreserved *surrender*. These are the nine

progressive steps in which the Indian scriptures envisage
the progress of the devotee.

If one can have relations with the Divine, relations
of devotion, if one can approach the Divine as one's
father, as one's mother, as one's great friend, it is
certainly legitimate—as Sri Aurobindo points out—to
address one's prayer to him and put forward before
him one's needs. Whether the needs are material,
psychological or spiritual, it matters little. All that
matters is that the child-soul needs, and the need is
formulated and transmitted to the Divine. He sanctions,
he who has promised that he sanctions and helps the
devotee to keep what is sanctioned.

How does the lever of prayer operate? In one
of the most beautiful explanations that he has given
—a rational explanation—Sri Aurobindo points out
that while it is true that there is a universal or a transcendental Will presiding over the creation, concerned
with its own large, massive objectives, it is also true
that it is not a mechanical, lifeless will. It is a personal
Will, taking account—at any rate as far as human
affairs are concerned—of the human will, the human
aspiration, and the human faith. Aspiration, faith and
will from the human end can move the Supreme Will
in its own favour. Of course it is left to the wisdom of
the Higher Will how it will respond, but it is possible
by prayer to move the Supreme will in one's favour.
How that Will will act and function, fulfil itself is
another matter which may or may not correspond
with what one expects it to do. But the fact remains
that human will, prayer has a certain effect of a pull
on the Supreme Will.

In the course of a number of explanations in
Savitri, Sri Aurobindo points out that when one prays

sincerely, he is linking his soul with the Divine through prayer. He says:

"A magic leverage suddenly is caught
That moves the veiled, ineffable, timeless Will...."
and in another place:

"A prayer, a master-act, a king-idea
Can link man's strength to a transcendent Force..."

Not all prayers are answered—we ourselves do not know what is ultimately good for us. That is why Sri Aurobindo observes somewhere else:

"Heaven's wiser Love rejects the mortal's prayer..."

Prayer is a powerful means of linking the human consciousness with the Divine Consciousness.

We have had hundreds of occasions where for over five decades we have had opportunities to contact the Divine in a human embodiment by means of prayer. Our prayers did not have to be transmitted through pen and paper; it was enough that a prayer rose in our hearts for the Mother to take cognisance of it, wherever she was, in whatever work she was engaged. We have often seen her, when she was signing documents, answering letters, suddenly halt for a second and then continue. She would explain that somebody had called—it may have been a call from Greece or from somebody in the Ashram, or from somebody in a hospital bed,—the call would reach her. And she also explained that whether her frontal consciousness took instant cognisance of it or not, the larger Consciousness embodied in her always responded. Prayer is an essential ingredient of the way of Love.

We have discussed the Fatherhood of God, the Motherhood of the Divine, the Divine as a Friend—these are all various gradations. The highest relation that it is possible for man to forge with God is one of love, utter love.

The Gita speaks of four classes of devotees, and says that all are legitimate. There are those who are distressed and seek succour—they are welcome. There are those who want their needs to be fulfilled—they are also attended to. There are those who want to know the Divine, acquire knowledge of the Divine—they are also welcomed. Finally, there are those who know the Divine and because they know, they love the Divine. For ultimately, the crown of Knowledge is Love. You can't but love when you know the Divine for what he is. You know that what the Divine is and what you are in your inmost being are but one.

This secret oneness is the fount of love. Whatever the motivation when one starts, as one develops these elements slowly drop off. There is even a stage when one becomes ashamed of the original motives and is intent on discarding them. And Love grows for its own sake. The lures of paradise—whether on earth or in heaven—do not last long. One does not seek the Divine to get even salvation, but only to love, to love more and still more.

There are one or two celebrated verses in Sanskrit spiritual literature which sum up the whole philosophy of the ultimate culmination of Love. It is a devotee who speaks to the Lord. He says:

"I do not bow down to your feet in order to arrive at the knowledge of oneness, nor do I offer my devotion to escape the fires of hell, nor do I want your favour to sport with the damsels or the nymphs of heaven, but I want to adore you, to wait upon you in the palace that is my heart, in state and state, in emotion and emotion."

How does such a man, who has no other interest except the love of God, lead his existence? What does he do when he has to eke out his livelihood? A famous teacher, who had realised the Divine, says in a memorable verse:

"Myself art Thou; my intelligence is Thy spouse, my life-energies are Thy attendants, my body is Thy home. All these enjoyments that I have in my life, they are Thy worship, and my sleep is my tranced concentration upon Thee. My walk is a circumambulation around Thee. All my words and speech are Thy praise. Whatever work I do, whatever action I do, all that, O Lord, is Thy adoration."

*   *   *

It is hard to break the spell with a question, but there is one. In the Katha Upanishad, speaking of prayer, Yama says, "For fear of Him...the sun hastens in his course and death too hastens in his course."

It belongs to that period in the evolution of human consciousness when one aspect of God was conceived as the ruler who had a law. There was a guardian of law for earth, another guardian of law for water, and so on. So that conception of God as the ordainer—not so much the protector as the keeper of law and righteousness—was still prominent.

Sri Aurobindo has pointed out in his *Foundations of Indian Culture* how the human consciousness had to move from gradation to gradation and it was only

after the mental heights were exhausted and the vital
regions traversed that the psychic and the deeper levels
came to the front and blossomed in that period of
mysticism and religion of love with Krishna, Radha,
Chaitanya, when the human soul learned to trust
God, to love God, and never to fear him. As long as
the human evolution had not freed itself from the unrege-
nerate animal heritage, this sort of compulsive ethics was
maintained.

So it served for...

The Supreme Diplomat, says Sri Aurobindo in
Savitri, uses even our fall for our rise. The Divine uses
even the devil for His own purposes. Fear is an intrusion,
but the Divine has used it to expedite...

*Incidentally, your rendition in Sanskrit of the Katha
Upanishad slokas was played in the Bharat Nivas...*

I see. A very powerful Upanishad. Sri Aurobindo
was fond of the Katha Upanishad. He has quoted
verses from there in so many places—in *The Future
Poetry*, in *The Foundations*, and in the earlier writings
particularly. And his explanations of the verses are very
original; they give a clue to what otherwise appears to
be a prosaic legend.

Speaking of the Way of Love, in one of his four
lectures on the Yogas, Swami Vivekananda summed
up all that the Indian tradition has to say on the subject.
These lectures were delivered in America and were
issued in separate volumes, and the yoga of devotion
was entitled *Bhakti Yoga*.

But even in India which is the home of Yoga and
all such movements, the living tradition of Love got
reduced to a lifeless system later, when they started

systematising it. Those who came after Chaitanya started classifying and dissecting all the emotions. They made the whole thing absolutely dry; that is the bane of systematising with the help of the intellect. Love is a thing which is to be felt, experienced, realised— not analysed by the mind. The moment the intellect enters into love, love ceases to be love. There is always a search for motivation. The psychologists are full of it, aren't they?

Can't the vital also have a motivation?

There is the pure vital, the real vital and there is a surface vital. When it is the true vital—what Sri Aurobindo calls the warrior of the Divine—there is nothing like it. When that vital catches flame, it is on its impulse that people give up their careers, give up even their lives, sacrificing themselves completely for love. It is from the inspiration, the impulsion of that vital that love derives its full strength for manifestation.

But can't love be expressed in the intellect too? In the mental-vital area?

It remains largely a theory like 'the world is one.' It is a concept of unity but as long as I intellectualise this concept, as long as I feel the oneness only in my mind without a corresponding effect in my consciousness elsewhere, it remains a mental theory. There are many philosophers who, at some time or other feel that the world is one, but they cannot communicate that truth to you. When you read their writings they do not make an impact and change the direction of your life, because they do not carry the participation of either the heart or the vital.

But still, love can come through a purified intellect, can't it?

Purified, yes. Because then intellect ceases to be merely the logical intellect and comes into its true role of reflecting the higher knowledge, then it reflects the true form of love.....and the true form of love in a purified mind is the perception of an intimate oneness.

But is true love really identified any more with the vital than it is with the intellect? Isn't it free of both, or the highest part of both?

Yes. The vital and mind are both intended to be instruments of the manifestation of love., once we purify them of their external dross.

The love that Jesus Christ released, for instance, on the earth, expressed itself on all levels of his being— his mind, his heart, his vitality, even his physical through healing. It was the power of love that healed; there was no magic or miracle-mongering in it. It was the love that brings wholeness and wholeness is healing.

But then, love is really no more a friend of the vital than it is of the intellect, is it? I get the idea that many people think, 'Use the feeling side, avoid the thinking.' But this is not necessary when the true being can use either instrument in its true way. Vital love is not really love. Neither one is really the Love itself.

I agree. Vital love is different from Love, because it is love that is appropriated by the vital. But when Love expresses itself through the vital, that is different.

5

THE WAY OF DEVOTION

Not long ago I read a book "*In the Days of Great Peace*". The author's name had been given as Mouni Sadhu. It was the name under which an Englishman, settled in Australia, had written an account of his stay with Ramana Maharshi at Tiruvannamalai. I had received the book for review, and as I read it I was so fascinated by it that I don't think I took more than two days to read the whole and write a long review article on it. I developed a great admiration for the author's understanding of Indian thought and his ability to communicate spiritual experience to the reader. And since then I was on the lookout for other books written by him.

The paper to which I sent the review was so satisfied with it that the next year when another book of the author—also published by Allen and Unwin— came out, they sent it to me for review. It was on "Concentration". With much anticipation I opened the book, but I was greatly disappointed, for after a handsome introduction to the subject, as soon as he began developing the theme the author started using numbers, diagrams, coloured points,—red, blue, white, green— to explain how concentration is to be done.

It looked ridiculous to me that an attempt should be made to explain a dynamic process like meditation or concentration in terms of numbers and dots. It can't be reduced to a system like that, it is not some kind of a physical science, but a movement, a psychological

4

process which can be indicated but can't be reduced
to numbers and systems.

Thereafter, I have come across more books by
the same gentleman, with the same handicap, same
disability. I have also found that other authors, who
normally write very well on other subjects, when it
comes to explaining certain lines of Indian yoga to
the western mind, try to reduce it to a system and in
the process fail to communicate the spark.

All this came to my mind, when I read again
Sri Aurobindo's yoga of devotion this morning, such
a subject cannot be reduced to a system as the psychological system of Rajayoga, or the physical system
of Hathayoga can be. It is a question of love, of
movement, of emotions; there is no set procedure
about it. It is something that wells up naturally, flows
out naturally, and there is no rule saying, "You can
go this way and not that way, follow this path and
not that path, go thus far and no farther". When
it concerns love—even in the human field—things
cannot be reduced to a system. Though there are
pathetic attempts by psychologists and psychoanalysts
to trace effect to cause and cause to effect, they are
only approximations, not clear accounts of what has
happened and what is likely or bound to happen.
There is always an imponderable factor when one
speaks of love; it depends upon the level from which
the love springs. If it is on the surface, you can explain
the motives, you can say what may be the reactions
to that love, whether it will be one of satisfaction or
dissatisfaction, whether it will be requited or un-
requited. But if the emotion is based deeper within,
there is no system of psychology or parapsychology

that can visualise in a fixed way the course that movement is going to take. We can speak of movements,
we can speak of phases in a broad way, but even there
when it concerns love, when it concerns devotion, one
cannot make water-tight compartments.

A certain phase may come earlier in some cases,
in others other phases may come earlier, but broadly
speaking, in the yoga of devotion, in which one seeks
to unite with the Divine through the path of love,
there are four broad movements. The first is the desire,
the quest of the soul for the Divine; second, the pain
of love unfulfilled, unresponded to, under struggle;
third, the joy of being possessed by the Divine Love—
one surrenders oneself absolutely: "whether you respond or not, my being stands surrendered to Thee"
is the spirit with which one surrenders. This third
movement leads inevitably to the fourth, the delight
of possessing the Divine. The culmination of the step
of being possessed by the Divine is to have the eternal
delight and bliss of possessing the Divine. But these
steps should not be regarded as inevitable procedures;
they are, broadly speaking, four movements.

The origins of the paths of love and devotion
are to be found in religions. Various religions have
attempted to forge the path to the Divine through
love. The first requisite is that there should be an
adoration of the Divine. One adores what is above, what
is around, and this process of adoration is organised,
given expression to, given shape in external worship.
This worship, as time passes, comes to be finally
woven into a system of ceremonial worship. Many
stop there; they feel satisfied once all the ritual of

worship is gone through. They feel that all is done. But it is not always so. After all, it is the inner adoration that gives soul to the body of external worship. In the Indian tradition, external worship is considered to be only the starting point. In the Tantras they have a broad categorisation of the classes of seekers. First comes the ordinary herdtype, the flock-type that just does what others do, they have not crossed beyond the animal level. Men of such type are led through external modes of worship. Then there is the heroic type that takes all things as they come and uses them as a means of communion with God. And lastly there is the godly type; such men are reminded by everything of God and look upon every thing as only a symbol of the Divine.

External worship is the first step; it is not a false or a wrong step. It is very fashionable among the votaries of the yoga of knowledge to dismiss external worship as sheer sentimentality. Sri Aurobindo has done great service in pointing out that external worship, external modes of expressing the inner emotion add a certain completeness to the procedure. On the physical plane it is the physical means of expression that stabilises, gives concrete shape to the inner relation and helps to establish it.

As one develops, as one worships,—remembering that the external worship must always be related to the inner adoration, that the inner adoration is the main thing,—the external worship gradually drops away or ceases to have the same importance. An inner adoration takes its place. And as this inner adoration takes root, no longer needing the stimulus of external worship and external ritual, the soul leaps up in adoration of the Divine. In whatever form one is used to, there is a natural and spontaneous flow of life, of thoughts, of emotions towards the Divine.

This turning of the whole life towards the Divine translates itself, when there is a modicum of sincerity, into a progressive consecration of life. There is a conscious attempt to surrender, to relate oneself at every step to the Divine whatever the work one may do, mental, physical or any other. At every step all is done as an offering of love to God, and as a result there grows a likeness to the Divine.

An important element of this discipline of self-consecration is purification. Certainly, by purification we do not mean external purification like bathing each time before one offers worship or sits for meditation—though one may certainly do it if one feels benefitted thereby—but a conscious remoulding of one's life by accepting only those elements which lead one a step closer to the Divine, and by eliminating those movements which retard one's progress. There is what is called a catharsis, a thorough washing-out of the impurities from one's psychological system so that the whole being transmutes itself into a temple where the Presence, attracted by the aspiration and the purity of the climate, installs itself. Ethical rules are applied in determining one's conduct by some, but in many cases what happens is that ethical perfection becomes an end in itself; it leads to a sort of self-complacency that one has arrived.

There are ethics and norms of different types, but the one barometer that is to be applied in all cases is whether this leads one nearer to the Divine, or away from the Divine. The first is good, the other is bad. The first promotes purity, the other promotes impurity. It is this way of self-purification, purification by catharsis,

cultivation of movements that build up one's nature
into the likeness of the Divine, that in the long run gives
what is called "liberation into likeness"—*sadharmya
mukti*. There are various types of liberations, but the
capital realisation of liberation into God comes when
our nature develops into a likeness with the Divine
Nature.

As in the other systems—psychological or psycho-
physical—here also there is the question of works and
there is the question of thoughts. It is comparatively
easy and it has been the tradition in many religions to
withdraw from this world of human relations, with its
many traps which are set by the enemies of God, by
Maya, to keep men tied down to this world which is a
huge snare. To withdraw into the forests or into the
lonely retreats of the heart, develop relations with the
Divine, and after establishing links, after living in the
divine largeness, to share one's experience with like-
minded devotees, lovers of God, is permissible, but
that is all. In movements like Buddhism, the sphere is
extended by including works of compassion, of charity,
of universal kindliness, as so many flowerings of the
spirit of love.

Certainly, this way is not open to the seeker of the
Integral Path. For us, the world is not a snare; the world
is a field of God. We have to play our part in opening
the field more and more completely to the play of the
Divine, and ourselves participate in the manifestation.
So, once we are awake to the breath of the divine love,
it is up to us to let that love rediate in our relations, in
our works, in our exertions in whatever field we act.
The whole world is looked upon as a body of God, and
with the same tenderness, with the same sincerity with

which one reaches one's love to God, one reaches out to God in humanity, in the world.

So also in thoughts. Thought-movements which lead us away from the central preoccupation with the Divine Beloved are put in the background and those that stimulate and create the mental climate favourable for the perception of divine oneness and divine love are encouraged and organised. In this process the remembrance and the repetition of a divine name, the use of a divine form have been found to be of capital value. A name is not just a label. Whatever it may have come to be in our way of life in the world, originally, in the proper scheme of things, a name uttered was something like a button which, when pressed, released into the atmosphere the powers, the qualities that are in the form bearing that name. The name is a symbol; a symbol of the reality it signifies.

So, if for instance, one repeats the name of Krishna, there is an immediate upsurge at the soul-level of delight. If one repeats the name of Shiva there is a release of silent peace. If one repeats the name of Mahakali there is a spread of dynamism, of power. We may not be aware, cognisant on our surface level, but in the inner realms, the moment a name is uttered with proper attention, what stands behind that name is evoked and it springs in life.

Similarly with form. A form is not just an outline given by human imagination or human caprice. The contents, the charge within take a particular shape in the subtle realm. According to the shape, one knows what is within. So each form answers to the content of truth that is in it.

That is why name and form have been given such great importance in Indian spiritual tradition. As happens in every human institution, these have lost their original power, but they can always be tapped and utilised. There have been cases where by sheer repetition of the Name, a link has been established with the Divine. Whatever the means—repetition of a name, evocation of a form, concentration on a form—there is an interchange, a link established with the Divine.

These are many different ways in which Indian tradition has, in a sense, pictured the growth of love. But, after all is said and done, there is one capital way, a most natural way, and that is the birth of love by itself. It is not that one decides, "I want to realise God and I shall do it through the way of devotion", and chooses the way of love. There are some in whom there is a spontaneous awakening of love; when the soul hears the flute calls of the Beloved it can no more be held back by the pleasures or the riches or the affluences of the flesh or matter. It insists on leaving aside all other considerations and calls, and follows the flute of the Divine Beloved. No rules, no conventions, no traditions can hold it back; the breath of divine love in such cases bloweth where it chooseth. There is a natural outflow, and the soul passions for God. There is such a consuming intensity of love that one wonders whether one is on the verge of lunacy.

A number of times the Mother has warned against condemning others of madness too easily. One never knows if it is a madness due to some damage of the brain or the result of certain imbalance caused in the system by an inability to establish a bridge between external nature and the inner growth. There is a divine madness that follows a period of pain, of separation, one struggles, one cries, but the Divine does not manifest himself, or if he does, it does not last long enough. There is a pain of separation, a cry of anguish, followed by repeated revelations of the Beloved till the whole system catches flame and one becomes one with the Divine Beloved.

Indian religion has presented this truth of the human soul turning to its Divine Beloved in picturesque language. It has taken all possible human relations and applied them to the love of the human soul for God. The most misunderstood has been the relation of God as the Lover. Many stories have been spread and misunderstood especially in the West. In India, certainly, nobody takes them literally, but in the West there is an insidious attempt to promote the cult of sex under the plea of the love of the human soul for God.

In the Mahabharata, the epic where Krishna and his work on earth are lauded, there is no mention of Radha, his beloved. Centuries later a cult grew up in India around Krishna as the divine Lover, and stories—naturally, built up around certain physical details—were woven into a whole epic called the *Bhagavata*. Poetic imagination is never wanting, particularly when it can be harnessed to vital needs, and scenes were conjured up in which Krishna was supposed to play the flute and call his nocturnal companions—the wives of poor cowherds—who left their husbands half-fed and rushed out to meet him under the moonlit skies and danced with him. Stories were told how, when these women were bathing in the river, Krishna stole their clothes and asked them to bare themselves before

him. Stories such as these are obviously grotesque. I
will tell you why. In the same epic when Krishna is
supposed to have sported and dallied with these damsels in moonlit nights for hours together, it is recorded
that he was then only nine years old! All those ladies were
housewives with husbands and children. How could
sex enter into the situation? Is it not apparent to the
meanest intelligence that the incident of removing the
clothes is just a symbol, a symbolic story of the human
soul undergoing the ritual of purification? The Lord
removes the vestures of desire, human emotions, and asks
the soul to bare itself to his sight, so that he may pour
his grace over it. This should be self-evident. Similarly,
can Krishna's marrying 16,000 wives be a human phenomenon? These wives of the cowherds, the Gopis, stand
for so many energies, so many human natures which
have been chained to the *purusha* in ignorance. God
comes to give deliverance to these human natures—
nature is always symbolised as female energy. It is this
fact of the advent of the Divine, through a special intervention, to give release to human souls, human natures
from thraldom to ignorance and animality, that is the
truth of the matter.

There is no mention of Radha as pictured in the
later books. It is a much later invention. Sri Aurobindo
describes Radha as a personification of human love
surrendered to the Divine. If Krishna symbolises and
embodies the Divine's Love for humanity, Radha
symbolises the love offered by the human soul to the
Divine in utter surrender.

After all is said and done, the true relationship
between the Mother-soul and the child-soul is one of
love. There is no question here whether one is a sinner

or a virtuous man, whether one is learned or stupid. All that matters is whether one can hold the cup of love and offer it to God.

    *   *   *   *

As no questions are forthcoming, I will end, stressing a point I made in passing. As I said in the beginning, the path of love has to be spontaneous. It is something which cannot be governed by logic nor can it be systematised or methodised. India is rightly regarded as the origin of this way of love, but it has also happened that in the later ages—particularly in Bengal— some schools of philosophy sprang up which tried to reduce the way of love into a fine system. Tomes after tomes have been written in Sanskrit, annotated, re-annotated still further by scholars, reducing the whole thing to a dry-as-dust philosophy. Time and again I have taken up these volumes but could never proceed beyond a page or two. Let me sound a note of warning— whenever you find anybody teaching how to culture love towards God, and making a system of it, beware of it. It has to be something spontaneous, you have to allow it to grow. All that you have to do is to support it, to build a climate in which it can sprout—what Mother calls a constant state of benevolence. She was never tired of repeating it: "Have benevolence for everyone, even for your enemy. Don't let your heart go dry or hard. The seed of love will not sprout on a barren soil. Don't be an ascetic—by all means reject inferior pleasures but don't reject life."

There has to be a broad acceptance of things, a constant state of benevolence in which one looks always to the favourable side of things, puts the most favourable interpretation on things, is much more charitable to others than to oneself. Thereby one creates a ground around oneself, within oneself, where the feet of the divine Beloved can step without being hurt.

Q. *I'd like to ask about the coming revolution in India.*

A. The question is about an article that has appeared in a local paper envisaging a general revolution in India. The author has said that this is the "Hour of God" of which Sri Aurobindo speaks, and people are asked to be ready. But that is not what Sri Aurobindo meant when he spoke of the Hour of God. He spoke of a spiritual manifestation and not a material revolution. It is easy for the author to think all the problems of India, or of the world, will be solved by a revolution. He has mistaken unrest, agitation for a revolutionary upsurge. What Sri Aurobindo wanted was a revolution in thought, a revolution in spirit, something of which the author of the article has no conception. He thinks only in terms of social and political changes. If spirituality can be of help in upsetting the existing social order, well and good, otherwise, he is prepared to upset even spirituality. This is the usual way of academic thinkers or disappointed politicians. The causes of today's unrest are not merely political, not simply due to social mismanagement, they lie much deeper. There is unrest everywhere, in every field, because of the inability or the unwillingness of man to respond to the pressure of the Time-Spirit to break out of his ego-shell, to universalise himself, before he can be ready to receive the transcendent consciousness in himself. The crux of the matter is that man should change. Unless individuals start changing their own lives, start forming collectivities promoting this change, this period of unrest will continue, and talk of impending revolution also will continue.

Q. *Do you think that we should accept everything from others with absolute forgiveness ?*

If one is concerned only with one's own spiritual development then this counsel of perfection—to treat everything that comes from others with absolute forgiveness—is commendable. But remember that the ultimate aim of Buddha was to withdraw from life; he was concerned to heal the wounds of life as much as possible, but the end was always to withdraw. But in a scheme, in a perspective which intends to build up life, to develop life into a picture of perfection, into a pattern of divine manifestation, one has necessarily to employ one's discrimination, see what are the elements of ill-will in another's reaction, what are the saving elements. One has to protect oneself from evil vibrations and encourage the good and the pure vibrations. One must note the wrong side of things but not allow it to determine one's attitude. One must note, one must send corrective vibrations—physical, psychological or spiritual—one must guard oneself against wrong ones and thus get on. It is a double labour; for a spiritual seeker who believes in the spiritual perfection of life, matters are more difficult than for a follower of Buddha.

6

THE DIVINE PERSONALITY

Our theme today is the question of the Divine Personality. For, as you know, it has been a long drawn-out battle among the philosophers whether personality or impersonality is the primal truth. Modern thought is generally one in pointing to a kind of impersonal force as being the author of the universe. There is an unmistakable tendency to reduce everything to some force—a force out of which everything issues. Even those who invest this force with some kind of consciousness or awareness point out that this consciousness expresses itself through a number of subsidiary forces, operates through a series of impersonal laws. This is the trend of modern thought.

Ancient thought also, starting from the other end—the end of the Spirit—, reduced everything to some ineffable Spirit. It went on to point out that this world and all its movements are derived, secondarily or even further, from an original impersonal Something which they would not name for want of an exact designating term. They simply called it "That".

Now this background is very disturbing to a devotee of God who likes to conceive of God in terms of a Person who listens to his prayers, who receives his offerings of love, who reveals himself to his soul. He is told by the philosophers of the path of knowledge that if that belief helps him, he may keep it. They imply that this belief in personality, in a divine Person, is a helpful crutch for the devotee to walk with till he acquires enough strength to face the truth that all that he was worshipping was only a mental fiction.

But, to the devotee, whatever be the conclusions of reason, whatever be the proofs of the logical intellect, nothing is more vivid, more real than the fact of the divine Person, around whom his whole life is organised. He has no patience with the arguments of the philosophers, who would prove to him that what the intellect perceives and determines is alone real, and not the weak sentiments of his heart.

To the integral seeker however, these two opposite approaches do not have much relevance for he depends neither upon his logical mind nor upon the effervescence of his emotional being for finding his way to the ultimate truth. It is his own spiritual experience and the authentic experience of those who have gone before him that are the standards by which he determines his life. To him the fact that his love, his devotion is accepted by Him or Her to whom he offers it is an incontrovertible fact. In fact he prefers to put aside the philosophical reason and mind as something irrelevant to him before the urgency and the vividness with which the personality of the Divine makes an impact on him.

Sri Aurobindo points out that in these matters neither the intellect nor the heart—as it functions— is enough. Both are guided by a superior faculty, intuition. We—each one of us—, whether we have that intuitive faculty functioning normally in us or not, have moments when we receive certain intuitive feelings or flashes which we first accept and later try to justify and explain to ourselves with the aid of the intellect or to have them corroborated by our experience. This intuition, which Sri Aurobindo describes elsewhere as

an arrow of truth, may reveal itself in any part of the
being. It may send its flashes to the intellect, or make its
warmth felt in the heart. The life-force has its own intuitive feelings, even the body has its intuitions. And the
experience of this intuition confirms the truth of personality.

When we look into ourselves, it does not need
much of a proof to understand or to realise that we are
not just a bundle of sensations, feelings, thoughts. We
also realise that we are not that bubble of ego which
centralises all these thoughts, feelings and movements
and gives us the illusion of a personality. And when we
look deep into ourselves, we realise that there is within
us an individual self whose shadow is the ego. Long
before thought and feeling can form, there is somebody there who projects the thought, whose thought
it is, whose feeling it is. So the fact of our personality
is anterior to the obvious fact of our thoughts and feelings
which are, comparatively speaking, impersonal. They
may center themselves around objects, but they are
impersonal movements, universal movements that pass
through ourselves.

The real factor that organises these universal and
impersonal movements around itself and grows on their
essence is the soul personality. The soul indeed has many
personalities. On each level of the being the soul, the
central being, projects itself. It projects itself as the mental
being, the emotional being, the vital being, the subtle-
physical being and the physical being. This is the truth
of each one of us and it is much more so with the Divine
Reality of which we are pale, incomplete reflections.

It is this perception of the reality of Person and
Personality in the Divine Existence that has led Indian

seers to speak of Brahman with personality and Brahman as the impersonal—in Sanskrit terms, the *saguna* Brahman and the *nirguna* Brahman. The *saguna* Brahman is the One with full personality, the whole universe is conceived as his body. He is picturesquely described in the Veda as the thousand-headed person, the cosmic person who projects one-fourth of himself in this universe while the rest of him transcends this creation.

What of the impersonal, one may ask. Adherents of the philosophy of *saguna* Brahman point out that the impersonal is the stuff out of which the person manifests. It is a formless, shapeless stuff from which the Divine builds so many personalities of himself. So without the person the impersonal has no practical consequence.

To this the champions of the impersonal point out that it is because the impersonal Reality is there that so many personalities can be projected. Personality is a consequence, is a formation of the impersonal. It is possible the personality may disappear, but that into which the personality disappears continues. It is by adopting this logic—incontrovertible when looked at by itself—that the philosophers, by successive elimination of forms, of personalities, arrived at three basic terms. They said that the ultimate Reality reduces itself to Existence, Consciousness and Bliss. Some went further and said that even Bliss cannot be included in the final impersonality because there are states of being where one does not realise or experience Bliss. Others then asserted that there are also states of being where one does not experience consciousness, so both Bliss and Consciousness were eliminated from the race towards the determination of the Ultimate, and only Existence, a

5

sense of *Being* remained. For without this sheer, ineffable Existence, there would be nothing to argue about and nobody to convince.

But this was not the end. It was left to Buddha to complete the logical process. He went a step further and asked why we say that existence is the final truth. We can as well conceive of a state when even the state of existence lapses into something which cannot be called existence. This is not imagination; in one's own quest of the self, quest of the truth inwards, one does have glimpses of a stage when the very conception of existence collapses. There are remarkable passages in the Epic *Savitri* by Sri Aurobindo where he describes the all-enveloping, all-swallowing states of the Nihil, the Zero, the nullity where nothing is. It is a Zero—may be an empty zero or a zero that is ineffable. Thus, the Buddhists, pursuing the path of the logical intellect, abolished even existence as the ultimate Truth.

Naturally, this sort of extreme position could not hold itself for long. Soon the question arose: existence but whose? There simply cannot be a state unless there is a being of which it is the state. So they again started and spoke of the Existent. If there is an existence, it is the existence of something, some reality. That reality is the Existent. And if this existent, this reality, this Real is conscious, this consciousness cannot just be a rarefied state of awareness. It is a dynamic state, it has a will of its own; it is out of this will that all projection comes to be. So they spoke of the Conscious Being. Then what about Delight? Because where there is consciousness, where there is a conscious existence, there is an ebullition of delight. So there, also, it was pointed out by those who had the experience, that Bliss is not just a state.

There is a Blissful Being, an Anandamaya Purusha who upholds the whole cosmos. The vibration of bliss, the movement of bliss proceeds from a Conscious Blissful Being.

All these aspects of the Existent, the Conscious Being, the Blissful Purusha, are concretised in the figure of Krishna in Indian philosophy. He is the Lord of Delight who accepts the love of the devotee. In the beginning different religions had different approaches to this conception of the Godhead. Originally they conceived of the Divine Person as a magnified edition of man. They endowed him with all the qualities of a human being, though on an exaggerated scale—caprice, anger, sense of justice, sense of righteousness. But in course of the development of consciousness and mind, certain difficulties came to be presented in the working of the universe. They had to account for many ungodly things that were taking place in the universe which could ill-square with their definition of the Godhead. Some philosophies erected the conception of the devil, on whose head they laid the blame for all that goes wrong in the universe, reserving for God the credit for all that is good. Some religions endowed man himself with the capacity to go counter to the will of God and start his career in sin. As maturity developed in the human mind, some devised the conception of Nature as being responsible for all that is uncomplimentary to God.

But looked at from a wider and larger standpoint, there is really no necessity to devise all these explanations to save God from the responsibility for all that goes wrong in the universe. In *The Life Divine* Sri Aurobindo points out how the whole problem changes its complexion

once one accepts the fact that the Divine is not something supracosmic, creating the universe and sitting
above it, watching what goes on, delivering judgment,
but a Reality which not only creates the universe, but
enters into it. In the Upanishads, it is clearly pointed
out, "Having created, He entered into it." He indwells
the universe, and of all that takes place it is He who
bears the burden. Whether in you or in me, in the animal or in the plant, it is the Divine that suffers, it is
the Divine that enjoys. We are only the outer instru-
mentations for the working, for effecting changes, for
the drawing of the sap of delight. Pain and pleasure are
only terms—negative and positive—of the experience
derived by God in the course of his manifestation.

The point is, the Divine is manifest in this universe
not merely as Force, not merely as Consciousness, but
as a Person, as a Personality who takes cognisance of
our needs, who accepts our offerings, who notes our aspi-
rations, and directs his Grace to us. That there is a
divine Person relating himself to each form, presiding over
each movement, gives meaning to every little movement
that takes place. If all was fathered, all was conducted
by some impersonal movement, some impersonal force,
what would be the meaning of human striving? Each
movement that man makes has a corresponding truth
in the Divine. What is the ultimate truth of Love? Is it
possible to love an impersonal Reality? One can contem-
plate, one can dwell in stillness on an impersonal Peace,
Calm, but Love cannot be still. Love is vibrant, Love
is dynamic. It insists on flowing towards its objective. Love is meaningless without the Beloved, and the
Beloved is irrelevant where there is no Lover.

The fact is both the personal and the impersonal
are aspects of the same Reality. From the human end

they are two gates opening on the same Divine Reality. Sri Aurobindo puts it picturesquely when he describes them as two wheels, two eternal wheels on which the human soul travels, parallel wheels which, opposed to human logic, but in pursuance of their own logic, do meet in Infinity.

If the mind in certain moods finds its summum bonum in an impersonal peace and silence, the heart also claims a rounded fulfilment for its emotions, for its stirrings of love, of self-giving, self-expansion, self-surrender. Around whom is this love to be organised if there be no Divine Person? Depending upon our approach the Divine reveals Himself, now as a Person, now as an impersonality. But in whichever way we come to experience the Divine, both are the truth.

Commonly, the Divine Impersonality is the truth for the Jnanin, for the seeker who follows the way of knowledge—at any rate in the beginning. But for the seeker who follows the way of devotion, the way of love, the Divine Personality is the all-sufficing truth. Even the worker on the path of Karmayoga—works— who starts originally with turning his will to the Divine Will, ultimately realises that the will is of the Lord of Works. Similarly, the seeker on the path of knowledge, after he grounds himself sufficiently well on the foundation of immutable, indefinable, ineffable silence and Peace, becomes aware that this Peace, this Calm is but a mood of the transcendent Being, whom the Gita calls the Purushottama.

As Sri Aurobindo points out, it is a capital contribution to the human thought positing the existence of the transcendent Purusha, in whom are reconciled the mobile and the immobile aspects, the dynamic and the

static, the impersonal and the personal. Both may appear
as contraries, but there is a level of consciousness, a
level of existence where both reveal themselves as com-
plementary truths reconciled in the totality of a transcendent Existent, Purushottama, for whom the personal and
the impersonal, the mobile and the immobile, the static
and the dynamic are terms of manifestation, polarities,
the two ends through which all manifestation has to
pass.

As far as the yoga of love is concerned, the Divine
Personality is the first truth, the truth of impersonality
can only be the background, the base. The Personality
is the fine flower which the human soul adores.

*   *   *   *

Q. *I was wondering if you could talk more about what
is called the higher Satchidananda and the lower Satchidananda?*

Actually the lower Satchidananda is a reflection of
the Higher Satchidananda in physical matter or in
life or in mind. It is described as experiencing Satchidananda at different levels. It is only a self-projection by
way of reflection. Only after the consciousness is built
up to cross the supramental belt does one come into
touch directly with the Being of Satchidananda. For
there it stands marshalled and organised on its move
towards manifestation. Here what we experience is a
reflected Satchidananda, there it is the original Satchidananda.

7

THE DELIGHT OF THE DIVINE

Before I start with the theme proper, "The Delight of the Divine", I think I should make a kind of a confession which will give you a clue to what led me to the acceptance of the truth of the delight of God. Ever since my childhood I always conceived of spiritual life as something austere, serious, solemn. I can't say what made me think that way, but I was not alone in this attitude— most of the spiritual traditions in India have it so. I am not very conversant with the mystic or spiritual traditions of the West. I grew up in the Indian tradition, looking upon spiritual life as something where one does not laugh overmuch or enjoy overmuch—in fact enjoyment is taboo—and since the aspiration to realise God, to see God face to face had been in a way implanted in me since childhood, in school and college I was always serious and was looked upon as a sort of kill-joy. Though all were not blunt enough to say that to me, still I knew they felt it. If my room-mates in the hostel planned going to the pictures I would say, 'No, I won't join', and I remember I derived a perverse satisfaction at having denied myself something and thereby thought to gain from the spiritual point of view. It didn't occur to me at that time that even to feel that I was denying myself gave me a secret satisfaction and boosted my ego. Be that as it may, I continued to feel and look serious, to look down upon those who habitually laughed, joked, enjoyed themselves going to picnics and pictures, playing games and in many other ways.

I was nineteen when I came here. When I first
saw the Mother my soul wept and wept, so much that
all those in the hall where the *pranām* function was going
on were moved and asked my mentor what had happened. He had a job explaining things to them. But that
was the last time I wept in that way, thereafter my soul
felt happy and started smiling. Suddenly I realised that
laughter, cheerfulness and joy were more natural and
brought one more into proximity with the Divine than
all the solemn seriousness that I could cultivate or summon.

I asked my teacher whether all that I had thought
was wrong because my experience here testified to the
contrary. He told me that it was not altogether wrong,
but I would know better as I grew up. And, indeed,
I have been learning every day that the truth lies neither
in complete solemnity and seriousness nor in constant
fun. Underneath the flow of Delight issuing from the
Divine, there is a profound awareness of the Truth.
The seriousness and the solemnity which certain traditions seem to foster make one detach oneself from in-
volvement in the petty rounds of the lower nature
and look to a deeper side of life. There is truth in both,
but the fact is that the easier door to the Divine is in
delight, in joy, rather than in dryness and solemnity.
Here again, there is Joy and joy, Delight and delight.
There is a delight which needs a cause, which thrives
as long as the cause is in operation—when the cause
is withdrawn, the delight dies. This is the vital joy, a
movement of the vital part in the being. But there
is an uncaused Joy, an uncaused Bliss which does
not depend upon outer stimulation; it is self-existent. The more one breaks out of the shell of self-cen-
tredness and opens oneself expansively, the more one

THE DELIGHT OF THE DIVINE

breathes the vibrations of Joy, of Felicity. The more one digs in and breaks through veil after veil of emotions entangled in ignorance and approaches nearer the soul—what Mother calls the psychic—the more one feels an outflow of bubbling joy. There is no apparent reason why it should be there, it is there and one just feels it.

The other day I was asked by a colleague why, when he woke up that morning he had a quiet happiness, a felicitous feeling. Obviously it was a psychic movement; if it had not been psychic, if it had been vital, he would have surely known what had stimulated it. As one finds one's natural base in the Divine within or the Divine around, the fount of Bliss opens up. That is because Bliss, Delight, Joy are inalienable characteristics of the Divine.

In yoga the aim, as we have seen, is the union of the soul with the Divine that exists, the Divine that is conscious, the Divine that is blissful. Human nature is progressively cultured and developed in its consciousness so that at first it reflects and thereafter it links itself with the higher, the Divine Nature. How it realises the Divine Nature depends upon the approach that it makes. If one thinks of the Divine as Peace, one eventually realises the Divine as Peace; if one thinks of the Divine as pure Consciousness, the Divine reveals itself as Consciousness; if one conceives of the Divine as Delight, the Divine reveals itself in waves of Delight. In fact, according to the approach is the response.

There is an old controversy in the Upanishads. These controversies will always be there as long as the human mind is at the stage of speculation. They speculate, for instance, whether Existence was earlier or Non-Existence. Then a seer in the Upanishad asks, "It is all very well to put this question, but how can Existence come out of Non-Existence? How can anything proceed out of nothing?" Similarly, in another context, one of the Upanishads declares that if one thinks of the Brahman, the Divine, as the Existent, one verily becomes the Existent. If one thinks of the Divine as Non-Existence, one ends up by becoming non-existent.

And that is after all what happened with the Buddhist philosophers. They started picturing—we do not know what exactly Buddha did, but the Buddhist philosophers started—thinking, conceiving and speaking of the Ultimate as a Nihil. And as they built themselves by spiritual discipline in the image of their ideal, they began to cancel themselves with the result that a successful culmination of their yogic life was to end themselves in a giant Nihilism.

The point is, as we conceive, as we approach the Divine, so will be the self-revelation of the Divine.

To the seeker of the Integral Yoga the Divine is not only conceived but also approached in all ways. The Divine is sought after in his conscious Existence through knowledge, the Divine sought after in his Power and Will through works, the Divine is sought after in his aspect of Delight through love, through devotion. Each way, each path, sets a certain objective before itself and pursues it through its characteristic means. There is the way of knowledge, there is the way of works, there is the way of love. But Sri Aurobindo points out that of all the ways, the way of love, the way of delight, is the most all-embracing. For when we approach the Divine through knowledge we inevitably start by separating ourselves from what we conceive to be not the Divine, we discriminate, we reject what in our tradition or in our view is not the Divine; we eliminate things, narrow our focus, and fix ourselves to our idea of what the Divine is. Gradually personalities, forms, individuals, lose their importance because we see them passing. We forget the truth that men pass but Man remains; hours and seconds pass but Time remains. So everywhere, in every field, as our power of discrimination works, we tend to eliminate from our vision forms and units, and our knowledge tends to become impersonal. But we cannot forget that the impersonal is not the whole of the Divine existence. There is also the personal aspect claiming our attention, demanding our allegiance.

Similarly in the way of works, we tune ourselves, we place our will in obedience to our ideal of the Divine Will—the Will of the Lord acting in the universe. We place ourselves as instruments and work in consecration. It is inevitable that once we start working in this way, once we bring in the concept of disinterested service and work, a certain attitude of detachment, of an impersonal instrument takes possession of us and the personal aspect is relegated to the background.

But in the way of delight things are different. Indeed there are religions that worship God as Delight, as Joy in order to arrive at the paradise of the joy of God. But a yogin does not take to the way of love to win anything for himself, he does not love God in order that God must love him. He does it for its own sake. As Mother once said, "One loves because one can't help but love." It is the nature of love to flow out. There is no calculation, there is no bargaining, one just loves because one has to love. With the Divine particularly, one pours out one's delight, one's joy, one's love at the feet of the Divine. That the Divine responds ten-fold is another matter, but one does not start in the yoga of love with an eye to the quantum of response from the Divine.

Pursued in this way, pursued with utter abandon, this way of love which takes on the character of the way of Delight, as it develops, brings about the culmi-nation of both the ways of knowledge and of works. As one loves and goes on loving more and more, one comes to know more and more of the Divine Being around whom the love is centered. The more one loves, the more one knows of the Divine; the more one knows, one realises that the Divine is one's own self. And one loves just as a fact, not as a discipline. Similarly, a God-lover does not, in this path, shut him-self always in ecstatic communion with his Beloved. Love demands to be expressed, it insists on radiating itself, pouring itself on those around in service, in works. Works come from one as scintillating radiations of love. One loves, not to get a purified will, not to get liberation, but because one has become an instrument, a loving instrument that cherishes the power of the Lord that courses through him. One is conscious that the force that works, the strength that sustains is of the Lord, of the Divine, and one throws oneself with utter aban-don in transmuting this energy of love into works.

So the way of love, at its depths and at its heights, reveals itself as the culmination of the way of know-ledge and of the way of works. Necessarily for an integral seeker, the Divine is not merely transcendent.

The Divine is present in the universe not less than in himself. The Divine is indeed present in the individual, he is present beyond but he is also present in the universe. The whole universe is looked upon and experienced as the Body of God. He sees that the same Divine who is at work in him is also at work in the universe, in the innumerable creatures that people the universe. The only difference is that he is aware, he is conscious that the Divine is active in him, is manifesting in him; the others are ignorant, unaware. In their egoism, in their limited vision they tend to think that they are acting. But the God-lover knows from where the hidden springs of life are moved, his vision sees what men in the universe do not and he tunes himself to the All-lover who plays in a million bodies.

That is not all. The fruit of Delight is love; one can experience love on the wings of Delight. It is Joy that leads to the source of love.

I am reminded of a reminiscence told by the Mother some 50 years ago. She said that this happened when she was twelve or thirteen. She was living with her grandmother who was a strict moralist and did not know at that time anything about physical love, love between man and woman. One day it so happened that some distant relations of her grandmother came to visit her at her home. When Mother entered the drawing room she found them—a boy and a girl—passionately kissing each other. This had no particular impact on the Mother. She said it was just like a scene in a film. She watched them and noted that they were deriving some joy in the process. As she was wondering about it, she suddenly felt an eruption of joy in herself and her whole being expanded. It was

only later that she came to know that what she had
experienced was the thrill of physical love.

Delight leads to love, true love. Love sees beauty
in what it loves. People are amused when a man calls
the woman he loves beautiful though she is quite ordinary, but behind it there is a great truth. One discovers
beauty because through love one establishes a link,
a certain identity which breaks through the surface
appearances. So to the God-lover, God is not only
present in the universe around but he is present as the
All-Beautiful. Everything puts on an appearance of
Beauty, one thrills to the presence of Beauty everywhere—maybe in a flower, maybe in an insect, an
animal. This is the acme of the Delight of the Divine,
to see the Divine as beauty at every level of creation.
To the extent that one is unable to appreciate beauty
in Nature, beauty in the universe, beauty in those
around, one is still in ignorance. As one grows, one
awakes to this omnipresent truth of the Divine as the
Beautiful.

                *   *   *   *

Q. *The Mother received visions of one whom she called
Krishna. How did the vision start, at what age, and in what
form was she taught?*

I believe it was when she was about sixteen or so.
She mentions that a number of spiritual teachers used to
come and give guidance to her during what she takes
care to describe as the 'body's sleep'. And of them there
was one person, one personality that came constantly
and she learned to call him 'Krishna'. When she saw
Sri Aurobindo for the first time, she recognised him as
the same 'Krishna'. And we all know that Sri Aurobindo
has close affinity with the Krishna of the Bhaga-

vadgita. He observed more than once that there was no difference between Krishna and himself. That is because the central Godhead that manifested at one time as Krishna now manifested as Sri Aurobindo. It had manifested earlier in time as someone else, even as it may manifest as someone else in time to come.

Q. *What would you say is the true meaning of the Mother meeting Sri Aurobindo on the physical plane?*

Obviously, Mother's meeting Sri Aurobindo on the physical plane meant the beginning of the manifestation that was intended in the present epoch of the new consciousness, the new truth. The Divine Consciousness that was to manifest descended, for purposes of manifestation, into two forms. It is an occult truth that wherever there is manifestation there has to be a polarity, there have to be two ends, two poises, the positive and the negative, the static and dynamic. This truth operated in human terms as a man in the East and a woman in the West, symbolising that both the East and the West have to come together to make the manifestation meaningful and complete.

The Mother observed once that her taking birth in France had a special meaning for she had to undergo a special education. Otherwise, everything in her was Indian. She often declared herself to be Indian first but she had to be born in the West in order to equip herself for the work with the best that western civilisation had to contribute.

Once all was ready—things had been revealed to Sri Aurobindo in terms of knowledge and his consciousness was ready, while the Mother's occult personality with all the power and spiritual consciousness embodied in her had matured—both came together. And

the first result was the starting of the *Arya,* which established in the human mind, for all time, the positive
ideals of human perfection and divine life. Sri Aurobindo
sought to work out this vision, this ideal in terms
of individual and collective perfection, applied it in
the different fields of life, and for six and a half years
this journal continued. A few years later the Ashram
started to form. The decisive starting point for the entire
project was on the twenty-ninth of March 1914, when
the Mother met Sri Aurobindo. And Sri Aurobindo
became convinced, on seeing Mother, that what he
had been seeking for—the complete surrender of the
human to the Divine, to the last cell—he had found
concretely realised in the Mother. And to the Mother,
the first sight of Sri Aurobindo was an assurance that
in spite of all appearances to the contrary, the hour
of liberation, the hour of salvation from ignorance
and inconscience was at hand.

                *   *   *   *

    The Mother is doing intensely what she had been
doing when she was in the physical body, but on a
larger canvas. Her work has spread out, become more
effective because in the subtler body, in which she is
functioning now, the Supramental Consciousness and
the Will and the Force are able to effectuate themselves more concretely than ever before. It is only certain distant results of this working on the subtler plane
that are glimpsed by some in their psychic experiences,
dreams or visions, or in their day-to-day life. But she
has been tremendously active, quickening the aspiration in everyone, assuring everyone of her present
·guidance in some form or the other. Each one feels
that she is specially present in him and for him, open-

ing up all avenues on earth that could possibly respond to the pressure of the higher consciousness, bringing into the open things that have to be weeded out, precipitating crisis after crisis so as to bring out what was hidden exposing untruths, uglinesses in order that they may be got rid of once for all, so that the hour of the divine manifestation may be brought nearer and nearer.

8

THE ANANDA BRAHMAN

All of you know about the Upanishads, which are not, as understood by Orientalists, speculations about truth, but records of ancient seekings for the Reality. There were seers who conducted their inner experiments to come into contact with the deepest or the widest reality they could conceive or experience, and they communicated their experience to the seekers of knowledge who gathered around them in their forest abodes. Probably the students took some kind of notes of those communications and it is fragments of those notes that have survived in what we call the Upanishads. That is why we see apparently disjointed portions and sudden appearances of new concepts, new thoughts. This does not mean that these seers were not capable of consistent reasoning or logical presentation. It only means that these are notes, transcriptions in an abbreviated form of the records of the inner pursuits of the sages.

In one of these ancient Upanishads there is a story relating how a young seeker, Bhrigu, approached his father Varuna, asking him to teach him what the Eternal is, what the Permanent is. The father asked him to seek That from which all things take their birth, in which all live, and into which all return in their passing. He asked him to apply his mind, to concentrate his energies and find it out. The son did accordingly and came back to his father with the report that he knew Food, or Matter, to be the Eternal. For, he said, it is from Food that all things are born, by Food they live, and into Food they pass. The father heard and then told him to go back and concentrate further. The son did accordingly, and when he came back next, reported that he had found that Life is the Eternal. Again he was given the same reply, and the boy concentrated again, and in the energy of his askesis, he found out that Mind is the Eternal. The father was still not satisfied, and sent him back on his mission. Once more he concentrated, came back and said that Knowledge is the Eternal. The father asked him to concentrate still further. Finally Bhrigu came back with his report that Bliss is the Eternal. For, he said, by Bliss are all things born, by Bliss all things live, and into Bliss they depart.

This is the ultimate; it is because of Bliss, an underlying Bliss that the creation holds itself together. In another passage of the same upanishad, the Taittiriya, the Bliss is spoken of in these words, "In the beginning all this Universe was Non-Existent and Unmanifest, from which this manifest Existence was born. Itself created itself; none other created it. Therefore they say of it the well and beautifully made. Lo, this that is well and beautifully made, verily, it is no other than the delight behind existence. When he has got him this delight, then it is that this creation becomes a thing of Bliss; for who could labour to draw in the breath or who could have strength to breathe it out, if there were not that Bliss in the heaven of his heart, the ether within his being?"

The Bliss is everywhere, it is all-pervading, but it is also inside man. It is inside the heart covered up by the toilings of the mind; it is there within the cave o the heart as it is overspread in the external ether.

Sri Aurobindo dwells upon this Bliss in a number of
passages in *Savitri*. He says:

> *A hidden Bliss is at the root of things.*
> *A mute Delight regards Time's countless works:*
> *To house God's joy in things Space gave wide room,*
> *To house God's joy in self our souls were born.*
> *This universe an old enchantment guards;*
> *Its objects are carved cups of World-Delight*
> *Whose charmed wine is some deep soul's rapture-drink,*
> *............*
>
> *Bliss is the secret stuff of all that lives,*
> *Even pain and grief are garbs of world-delight,*
> *It hides behind thy sorrow and thy cry.........*
> *Indifference, pain and joy, a triple disguise,*
> *Attire of the rapturous Dancer in the ways,*
> *Withhold from thee the body of God's bliss......*
> *A vast disguise conceals the Eternal's Bliss.*

The underlying idea in the passage from the Upanishads,
or the lines from *Savitri*, is that the Eternal, the Ineffable is present everywhere as Bliss. If we are not aware
of it, it is because we are too far lost in our petty surface
preoccupations—jumpings of vital desires, monkeyings
of the mind, inert habits of the body — to perceive that
there is a stress of Delight running through the universe.
Sri Aurobindo observes in *The Life Divine* that in spite
of all the pains and sorrows of the world, there is still
the will to live, man still wants to live. That is because
the total of joy is always more than the total of pain;
otherwise the will to live would not be there.

This—the Eternal as Bliss—is what they call the
Ananda Brahman, Brahman as Ananda. We have discussed and studied Brahman as knowledge, Brahman
as power, Brahman as light; now we come to Brahman

as delight—a multi-faceted delight, at the ebullition of which the universe has come to be, and due to the streaming of which the universe continues and furthers its course. Even among those who do not claim to live a spiritual life, to be doing yoga, many have had perceptions of this impersonal joy, uncaused Delight in the world. Suddenly we awake at certain moments to an impersonal joy. There is nothing that has happened specially that we should be joyous about, but we breathe an air of delight, we respond to some call of joy in the universe. That is because there is this Bliss as the secret ether in the universe. And, as we observed, it is also there in the heart of all creatures. It may reveal itself to some as beauty, as beautiful forms and patterns as beauty of sound, as beauty of existence. Those whose aesthetic being is more developed have perception of this existence of Delight in the form of Beauty. There are those whose aesthetic being may not be developed, but whose emotional being is, who are touched by some psychic ray. They awake to a univerasl sense of compassion and love. For no apparent reason they are flooded with a spontaneous movement of goodwill, kindliness, helpfulness, a love for all creatures which has no element of calculation in it. These are all outflowings from the Ananda Brahman and a seeker of the path of love aims to approach and realise this Delight Brahman in all its ways of being, in all its possible ways of relations. But because the human mind is confined, it needs to culture itself, to purify itself before it can put itself in tune with this Eternal Bliss. It is one thing to have a sudden experience, to open for a few moments to this transmuting experience, which may even change the whole life and another thing to have the experience permanently. For that the being has to completely reverse itself from its normal direction and absorb and assimilate into itself the Bliss aspect of the Eternal. It has to universalise itself. No human mind, no human soul can embody, receive and hold within itself this Eternal Delight, unless it breaks out of its shell of ego and starts universalising itself. It is a flow that refuses to be checked. When we change its form, we deform it into human pain; it is in this sense that human pleasure and pain are limitations and deformations of the Divine Bliss.

There are, Sri Aurobindo says, three ways in which the Bliss Infinite, this blissful Existence, reveals itself. It can reveal itself within us, around us, above us. Within is of more importance to us, because our way is essentially an inner way, though not exclusively that. Within ourselves there are two centres from where the Eternal Bliss can reveal itself. One is the centre in the heart where the *purusha* of the heart presides. From there, when the Bliss manifests, it comes in uncontrollable movements of love, expansiveness, joy and it floods the being. The external being may even lose its balance unless it is strong, well balanced and organised. When this outflow starts from the heart centre, it spreads over the whole being and it has to be disciplined to find its right expression in external movements. It shoots up into the head, it tries to shoot up to its transcendental source, soaks the mind and casts its thoughts in its own stuff, so that the mind thinks of nothing but love and of surrender of itself in love. There is also the centre in the head where the *purusha* is seated, in the language of the Tantra, in the thousand-petalled lotus, from where flow down the Divine energy and the light and the Delight. The Divine Delight appears first as peace and when the peace is stablised, Delight courses in endless streams.

Here also, an experience does not mean a realisation. One may get an experience of this flow from the head centre, but it is only a beginning. The flow has to be organised, systematised and the various parts of the being made receptive to the flow of that Ananda so that the whole being is inundated with the downpour of Bliss. Thus does the ineffable Delight reveal itself from within.

For some it may reveal itself in the universe around; suddenly it may so happen that the various forms that one sees reveal what is behind them. They glow with a new life and each form impinges upon one with its charge of delight. The whole world appears to be a festival and what normally acts as a veil to truth, loses its opacity and becomes a symbol for the Beauty and the Delight of God. It is then that the Delight in the universe is manifested and the person who experiences it can see no ugliness, no division because his consciousness is aware only of Harmony, of Beauty, of Delight.

One may realise this Delight Brahman as something high above. One opens oneself by aspiration and by a consistent surrender, until one evokes the higher Delight, and the wine of the Immortal courses in the veins. First there is actually a physical sensation of ice-cold drops falling drop by drop from above. Thereafter there is a flow. But, Sri Aurobindo points out, it is not enough to receive the flow, one has to assimilate it, one has to re-mould the whole being in the image of the Delight, in the stuff of the Delight and forge a bridge between oneself and the super-conscient Delight.

All the three revelations—the revelation within, the revelation around, the revelation above—are inter-related. Some of the traditional yogas are satisfied with the realisation of this Delight in one part of the being, in one section and they call it liberation. But for the integral seeker that can only be a starting point. He has to realise the Divine Being in all its ways of being. Even if he starts with knowledge, it has to be suffused with love so that the union is a luminous union. If he starts with works, it has to be an active union; if he starts with love, it has to be an ecstatic union. All the three have to be combined, integrated so that ultimately—and this is the speciality of Mother's and Sri Aurobindo's teachings—, simultaneously, at different levels of the being, these different unions with the Divine can operate. He can be in tune and in union with the Divine at the plane of knowledge in a luminous way, at the plane of will and action in a dynamic way, at the depth of the psychic in a sweet and blissful way. All the three are possible and if he has a comprehensive pers-pective, it is possible to integrate all the three realisations.

*   *   *   *

One of the Mother's classic formulations of Divine Truth in manifestation is the truth of the four-fold revelation of the Divine. She says that the Divine re-veals itself in the mind as knowledge, in the vital or will as power, in the heart as love and bliss, in the body as beauty of form. This tallies very much with Sri Aurobindo's observation that Beauty is the priestess of Delight, Beauty interprets Delight. There cannot be Beauty unless there is Bliss behind it. Many of us stop with the enjoyment of the beauty of a form, we stop at the aesthetic level. But if we concentrate a little deeper, if we remain quiet and allow that beauty to grow in us, we awake to the Bliss or the Delight behind that has caused that beautiful form to come into existence. What delight a painter must have when he creates a beautiful painting or a poet when he composes a beautiful poem!

The ultimate truth of all things and movements in this manifested universe is Delight; for it is out of Delight that the Divine has manifested, and he is still deriving Delight through all the experiences that the world is going through, and it is towards some consummation of Delight that the world is being led. Delight is the beginning, Delight is the middle and Delight is the end.

If Delight is the nature of this existence— Sri Aurobindo asks himself in one of the chapters of *The Life Divine*—Why is it that you and I don't feel life as delightful as it is described by philosophers and saints, why is it that we see so much misery, undergo so much of suffering every day? He analyses the problem in two chapters: *Delight of Existence, the Problem and Delight of existence, the Solution,* and shows that the crux of the problem is in self-limitation; due to ignorance, the hold of the inconscience or for whatever reason, we limit ourselves, we narrow ourselves within our ego bounds. And it is because our life-force, our life-personality is so narrowed down that it cannot bear the waves of universal life when they beat upon it. It shrinks. Each shrinking is a movement of pain. When it can bear it somewhat, it is a movement of what we call pleasure. But both are imperfect and wrong responses. If this wall of limitation is removed, if these barriers are thrown open, if we can face and front the cosmic waves

of life and mind as they come upon us, then Delight
answers to Delight and all becomes a sea of Bliss. So
the first and the most important thing to be done is to
liberate ourselves from the self-imposed bondage of the
ego.

The ego is not merely a philosophical concept. There
is an ego of the body, there is an ego of the life-force,
there is an ego of the mind, there is an ego of the emotions and an ego even of the spiritual kind. Each ego
has to be consistently broken, and the last ego to be
broken, as the Mother once humourously said, is the
ego of spirituality. That I am spiritual, superior to
others, different from others is the last spiritual ego
that has to be broken asunder. It is only when one
universalises oneself and becomes a cosmic man that
one earns the right to breathe eternally the air of Delight.

Q. *It is my own experience that it is so limitless, this
tremendous expansion and somehow one wants to find somewhere in it something to hook on to...*

Concluding the chapter, Srı Aurobindo points out
that the acme, the crowning step of this impersonal,
ineffable Delight comes when we realise that it is a
way of being of Him who is the eternal Lover, who is
the Eternal, the Beautiful, the Lord and Master of
our being; the impersonal Love, the limitless Delight
are the ways of being of One to whom we are linked,
whom we take to our bosom. It is then that the acme
of Delight is realised between the lover and the Beloved. The ultimate Truth according to Sri Aurobindo,
and according to the highest mystical experience
recorded, is of the Divine as the Lover and the Master.

Q. *How should one deal with physical pain?*

First you have to meet it on the human level by endurance. Don't run away from pain but endure, summon all the strength that you have and endure. As you learn to endure, you detach the mind from it and introduce the element of indifference—whether there is pain or no pain, let the soul be indifferent. Thereafter, when you have realised enough to detach the being from the suffering, learn to bear it without shaking, it is to be offered to the Divine and in the measure in which the consecration, the surrender of the being is made, the impact of the pain becomes less. And slowly, the other face of pain which is one of joy starts revealing itself and the experience leads ultimately to a movement in which what strikes the frontal being as pain is rendered in terms of joy, of ecstasy of the soul. For to the awakened soul pain and pleasure are only means of deriving the necessary experience for its growth. We can have some idea of this happening if we picture to ourselves how a patriot, a hero on a battlefield, even when he is being physically wounded or tortured, the body subjected to untold sufferings, can feel joy, how his inner being can be aglow. It feels the joy of fulfilment even on the physical plane. So at the spiritual level it is possible by gaining endurance, indifference, detachment and surrender to the Divine, to have all experience transmuted into one of joy.

Q. *That answer that you just gave is very intersting because many people in the Ashram, in casual conversation say that when they have some pain they immediately offer it to Mother, they don't go through the previous steps you spoke about. And I am sure that offering it to Mother is better than what they might normally do with it, but it raises the interesting question of what kind of growth they might be missing by not going through these other steps.*

One doesn't grow, pain and suffering don't serve the purpose for which they are given. One just makes use of a facility that is given. It can be used till one gets a foothold, but thereafter one has to learn the hard way, otherwise it does not become part of one's spiritual conquest. That part remains where it is. It is just like my committing to memory a poem and reciting it by memory to the teacher without understanding it and another studying it part by part, liking it, making it part of himself and then reciting it. So spiritually, it is the hard way by which one has to learn.

Q. *When you say one only learns by hard knocks...*

A. Hard way, not necessarily hard knocks. When I was learning physical exercises, it was dinned into me that if I wanted to develop my muscles, I must do exercises the hard way. Then only, the time spent in physical exercises will have been worthwhile. One can always go through the movements, but whether one does it the hard way, that's another thing. Knocks are not an indispensable part of spiritual life—not at all—but people often invite them.

9

THE MYSTERY OF LOVE

We have been studying the yoga of love and have now arrived at a point where we can take stock of the advantages and the excellences of this way of approach to God over others. We can conceive of a large number of seekers who are not mentally developed enough to tread the path of knowledge; we can also conceive of many who are unable to use their will or develop their will as required for a ceaseless consecration of works to God. But there could hardly be any who do not know how to love—life and love go together. Everyone, whatever his development, knows spontaneously, instinctively to love. It does not matter what the quality of this love is, to what extent this love is egoistic or self-regarding; the fact that there is this capacity for love in a human being is enough. One can always start from where one is. Even if the love is self-regarding in the beginning, its character can change with time.

It is in this spirit that Sri Krishna lists among his legitimate devotees—he speaks of four kinds—those who seek him out of distress, those who seek him in order to gain objects of desire, those who seek to know him and finally those who know him and love him because they know him.

It is an ascetic superstition that a seeker of God should not pray for the fulfilment of his desires. It is because one has trust, one has confidence in the Godhead—whether one conceives of the Godhead as the Father, the Lord or the Mother—that one approaches it with a childlike attitude. And it is the law of spiritual dynamics that the Mother-soul always welcomes the child-soul on whatever plea. Even a prayer to God with trust for the granting of certain wishes or desires forges a link and the very granting of these desires—which God always does, provided it does not go against the real interests of the seeker—opens up an avenue for the growth of love. There have been a number of instances of people who started with desires, but later on with their becoming ashamed of this motivation, the lower elements simply dropped off.

This then is the easiest and the most accessible path of all—the way of love. There is a belief among the intellegentsia and the philosophers that love for God in a personal form is an inferior movement, whereas love for the impersonal divinity is a higher one. Indian tradition does not support this view. It is argued by those philosophers that when one loves the divine Impersonality, the human personality ultimately merges itself in it and is no more—there is neither the lover nor the loved, there is only love.

This sounds very well in words, but in practice it is different. Even when one starts thinking that the impersonal Divinity is a status of being, a state of existence, the question arises, "Is the existence an inert existence or has it a consciousness of its own?" It is conceded by all that the supreme Existence that is conscious and blissful is only a way of positing an Existent, a supreme Being that is conscious and is blissful. This consciousness, again, has power—it is not inert. And this power of consciousness, or more properly this consciousness as power, is called Shakti in Indian terminology. All the universe is a projection, an emanation from this Being, from this power. And this Being lends itself to all types of relations with the human soul.

Even when one conceives theoretically of the possibility of the human adorer being lost in adoration—neither the lover nor the beloved being there any more—one should remember that this is only the acme of experience; it is not a permanent state. The individual adorer, the lover, the human lover exists—may be in the bosom of the Infinite, of the Ineffable Being, but he exists. The Being exists to receive and respond. The state of union, the state where there is only one, is a crown of achievement but at no time does it cancel the fact of the existence of the individual.

I remember the Mother saying that if it was the Divine intention that the individual soul has at some time to cancel itself out of existence, to disappear into the bosom of the Infinite, it would not have been projected at all. The very fact that an individual soul has been emanated shows that a particular stress in the oceanic Being of God wanted to manifest itself, to manifest the glory of the parent Divine, and it will continue to do that, whatever the type of intermediate experience. The individuality, the fact of the individual existence of a soul cannot be cancelled. The person who loves is the individual, the person who gets the experience of unity is, again, the individual. And after the consummation of that experience, it is the individual who continues, who remembers and who cherishes that experience.

The Godhead of which all impersonal existence is a state of being is the ideal of the practitioner of the yoga of love. It is not possible to realise the full extent of this being of Godhead immediately. As the individual

grows, so grows and so extends the Being of Godhead
that reveals itself to him. That is the law of evolution—
as one develops, as one grows, the capacity to receive,
to understand, to embrace becomes more and more.
The mind, the emotions, the will, all the three have to
be sedulously cultivated and trained to share in this union
of love, in this outpouring of love, in this reception of
love at their respective levels—the level of knowledge,
the level of emotions, the heart, the level of will. It is
to provide for this inability of the human consciousness
to grasp all at once the full glory of the divine Being
that the Divine reveals himself in the form in which the
adorer approaches him.

He reveals himself, he is celebrated in terms of
the absolute of certain qualities, certain powers to
which the human consciousness is open. That is what
we call in India the Ishta Devata or the Godhead-
elect of human nature. Each nature has its own conception of the form in which it would like to approach and
realise the Godhead, it has got its own temperament
and nature which can respond only to identical formulations of the Godhead. There are various forms in
which the Divine Godhead has manifested itself—what
we call Krishna, Shiva, Vishnu and so on. Each of these
Godheads is a formulation of particular qualities,
powers, functions or principles of the Divinity. The aim
of the integral seeker is to synthesise all these modes of
manifestation of God. He has to know that there is no
real conflict between these several self-presentations or
self-formulations of the Godhead. They are functional
manifestations at certain junctures of human development. The seeker attemps to *personalise* a select form of
the Godhead by building an all-embracing relation. He
is not content to experience the Godhead whom he

adores in his own chosen forms; he seeks to realise this Godhead also in other forms.

First, one realises that the Beloved is present in oneself. One may start with a mental conviction, based or not based upon experience but upon faith. One dwells upon it, one concentrates upon it, and if one has the grace of God operative directly or through an appointed teacher—not self-appointed teachers, but God-appointed ones—then one gradually becomes conscious of something within oneself at the deepest core of one's being, which is different from the rest of oneself. There, seated within the heart—the heart-cave, to use the classic expression of the Upanishads—is the Godhead, there the Lord is seated. One starts with that conception and with good luck, the help of holy company, askesis, meditation, prayer, concentration, one arrives at the perception of the Godhead.

But it is not enough, it is only the first practical step. After one is convinced practically that there is the Beloved—the Divine Lord—within, one has to proceed to organise the whole of one's life around him. It will not do to enter into communion with him only in special periods of concentration or worship or meditation. One has to open up all the regions of the being one by one—the mind, the heart, the life-energies—and the easiest way to open them and bring them under the rule of the inner ruler is to cultivate the habit of not doing anything, of not acting or reacting to any situation without reference to the Divine within. In the beginning one may be misled, one may think that one has referred, but the very sincerity of the seeker ultimately tells and draws forth the inmost response. The whole of life becomes a movement proceeding with the sanction of the Lord within.

7

Similarly, there are those who start with work as their means to union. The seeker begins to work for the God he loves, as a servant of God. He tries to see what God wants of him, and with utmost sincerity he does the work he feels has devolved upon him. This is the first step, the lowest step for the God-lover in the way of works. Gradually, as his will develops and subordinates itself to the higher or the deeper will of God, he becomes an instrument of God. That is the second step; from being a servant of God he evolves into an instrument of God. To use a classic similie, he is a string on the harp of life played by God. He gives forth only those notes that are played by the Divine. As the identification as the instrument grows, he comes to a point when he has no separate existence even as an instrument. He becomes just a slave of God. What God wills, is automatically effectuated. There is an immediacy of union. There is no gulf as between a master and a servant or between something that impels and the instrument that transmits. There is at this level of work a complete identity between the Master and the worker.

Similarly, in the yoga of love, narrow conceptions, philosophical formulas turn out to be absolutely inadequate. After all, as Sri Aurobindo points out, how can the human tongue in its poor speech speak of those ineffable sweetnesses, those innumerable touches of love supreme? The Divine Godhead, the Divine Lover reveals himself in a thousand ways. One never knows how he will come or where he may be seen. It may be that when you look around, you have the sight of an ideal face, a heroic mould and something in you catches fire. You look at a beautiful building, a temple tower, the blue sea or a beautifully carved image and you are filled with delight at the infinite expressions of the Divinity. The Divine Godhead reveals himself as a master, as a friend and comrade who shares your joys and your pains; he is the charioteer of your chariot of life guiding you, comforting you, surprising you at odd moments with his glory. You never know where and when you may stumble upon the Godhead when you have love for God in the heart. In the beginning you may not be aware on the surface of the Divine Love which is waiting to manifest; you may be lost in petty activities or lost in the pursuit of human love, but very often it happens that the human love after a certain point becomes a gate opening on the vastness of the Divine Love.

Many of you may have heard the real life story of one of the celebrated saints of India, Tulsi Das. He was a poor man but a learned brahmin, as all brahmins were in those memorable days. His head was always loaded with the scriptures, he could solve the most intricate and profound problems of philosophical import but he was very much attached to his wife. He loved her more than anything else. One day Tulsi's wife had gone to her mother's house across the river. That night Tulsi could not contain himself. He wanted to be with his wife. He swam mile after mile of the river at midnight when it was pouring in torrents and reached the house of his wife's parents. But she was on the upper storey and he did not know how to get in as doors were closed. Just then in that darkness his hands felt what seemed to be a long rope and using it he climbed up to his wife's room. His wife got up and seeing him was amazed that he had come in that foul weather in search of her. She asked him, "How did you come?" He said that he had found a rope. When she looked, she saw it was no rope but a serpent! Then she was moved to say to her husband, "If you had loved your Rama with half the love that you are bestowing on me, you would have realised Him." Her words shot like arrows into his heart and he forthwith climbed down the window and went away never to turn back. Today he is known as the foremost devotee of Lord Rama who as you know was an incarnation of the supreme Godhead.

Many are the stories and legends of how the Lord, the Divine Beloved reveals himself to erring humanity not only as a friend, not only as a comrade but even as an enemy. When one approaches him as an enemy, one hates him but in the very process of hating one concentrates all one's consciousness on that object of hatred, and that object suddenly reveals itself to be the Divine Lover. There are a thousand and one gates to the Divine Beloved. He is not only the pursued but is also the pursuer.

I do not know how many of you have read *The Hound of Heaven* where there is a vivid and graphic description of how the Grace of God pursues man, pursues his soul through all the alleys, through all its erring detours, until it overtakes him. In Sanskrit the word for Grace is *anugraha* which means "that which pursues and holds". Man may try to run away from the Grace but the Grace being what it is pursues and catches him in a hook from which there is no escape. Of course it is a question of how many lives it takes to be caught by the hook of Grace.

That man pursues God is one side of the matter, the other side and one that is more true is that the Grace of God, the Love of God, pursues man. It is because God loves that man is at all able to love God, otherwise man would always be lost in the petty preoccupations of egoistic pursuits. Because there is a call from within, there is a constant downpour of Grace from above whether we are aware of it or not; one day we wake up to this fact of love and then we wonder how we could have failed to notice the presence of God everywhere, failed to sense the flow of God's love in our veins.

Such is the divine love and the crown of this love is liberation—not individual liberation somewhere into a beyond—but a liberation into a state of union with God, with the Beloved. And this union of love includes in itself all other unions that are achievable by the paths of knowledge, works and other ways. When there is absolute union between the human soul and the Divine Beloved, between the seeker and the Lord, there is automatically a closeness—what is called *samipya*, *salokya*, liberation into nearness, liberation into 'like world'. Similarly there is so much of identity that each reflects the other so that at times it is difficult to say who is the human and who is the Divine; there is such a likeness between the adorer and the adored, it is called *sadrishya*, the likeness—this is another type of *mukti*, liberation. All these—the liberation into likeness, the liberation into proximity, the liberation into sharing the same world—these are constituent parts of the absolute union obtainable by the divine love. That is why Sri Aurobindo says that the divine love is the secret of secrets, the mystery of mysteries.

*   *   *   *

Q. *There was somebody who came to the Ashram after having read Sri Aurobindo's books for 20 or 25 years... and after two weeks he decided he would get back. And he thought he understood Sri Aurobindo because he had been reading him for so many years and his understanding was that he came here*

*to transform India from a place of poverty into a prosperous
country and he came to the yoga because he thought that was the
work, social transformation. And then he saw the Mother and
said, "Well, all I saw was an old lady". He felt there could
not be anything more because if there was he would have felt
it. I said to him: "If you don't see something, maybe that is
because you're resisting it". And he replied "St. Paul was
full of resistance but then God struck him". When he said that
it made me think that maybe that's what God did with St.
Paul when he turned himself into an object of hatred. St. Paul
was full of venom and was persecuting Christians. I just won-
dered if you could say something.*

Obviously his activity of persecution of those
devoted to Christ was his last resistance, his way of
fighting the Grace that was coming to him. He may
not have been fully aware at the conscious level of his
mind, but he had been chosen. The ignorant part of
him, however, was fighting it to save itself from being
engulfed by the Divine Consciousness. Usually such
intense hatred, such intense feelings are the last con-
vulsive movements of a dying resistance.

Indian mythology is full of such incidents, of
course with typical exaggeration common to the Pura-
nas. Some devotees had deliberately chosen to be born
as enemies of God rather than as devotees, because
they said that way their salvation would be quicker,
—because God would pay more attention to them. The
truth behind these stories is that when evil or false-
hood presents itself in an extreme form, it calls forth a
radical elimination from the Divine, it is not allowed
to work its way out, it is struck off the cosmic lists.
It is only a way of saying that even when we see the
maximisation of evil, somewhere lurking there is the

solution. It is deliberately allowed to gather itself so that at one blow it can be eliminated.

Even in medical science certain poisons are encouraged to accumulate in one part of the body as in boils, so that one can eliminate them more effectively. Certain diseases are of that type, so that the whole system may be rid of them. Ultimately from this point of view, the Divine Love is at the bottom of all movements. The whole movement of the evolution of the earth from the state of unconsciousness onwards has been possible because of that single ray of Love which came straight from the Supreme in answer to this creation which got involved in complete darkness of Nescience at the nadir of devolution. And it is that Love which sees to it that despite all deformations and perversions, the movement is Godward. Even the so-called atheists and agnostics also serve the Divine Love without knowing it. They won't admit it, of course.

Perhaps you know that when China attacked India and the Mother went in her subtle body to see what could be done to stop the war and increase the pressure of the forces of peace and harmony, she saw that all were closed to the Divine vibrations and the only people who were receptive to the Divine suggestion were the Chinese! Nobody has been able to explain why the Chinese chose to go back at the very hour of their victory. The truth, perhaps, is behind the surface events.

That is the character of love. It acts whether the recipient is aware of it or not, whether the recipient responds or not.

Other Titles by Sri M.P. Pandit:

Occult Lines Behind Life	$3.95
Sadhana in Sri Aurobindo's Yoga	$3.95
Dhyana (Meditation)	$1.95
Japa (Mantra Yoga)	$1.95
Gems from the Gita	$3.95
Gems from the Veda	$3.95
Mystic Approach to the Veda and Upanishads	$4.00
Studies in the Tantras and the Veda	$3.95
Upanishads: Gateways of Knowledge	$4.00
Yoga for the Modern Man	$4.00
Yoga in Sri Aurobindo's Epic *SAVITRI*	$7.95
Yoga of Works	$8.00
Yoga of Knowledge	$5.95

available from:
your local bookseller or:

LOTUS LIGHT
P. O. Box 2
Wilmot, WI   53192 USA
414-862-6968